The 9 Truths
about Weight Loss

DANIEL KIRSCHENBAUM, Ph.D.

THE

9 Truths

about

WEIGHT LOSS

The No-Tricks, No-Nonsense Plan
for Lifelong Weight Control

❖

HENRY HOLT AND COMPANY • NEW YORK

Henry Holt and Company, LLC
Publishers since 1866
115 West 18th Street
New York, New York 10011

Henry Holt® is a registered
trademark of Henry Holt and Company, LLC.

Published in Canada by Fitzhenry & Whiteside Ltd.,
195 Allstate Parkway, Markham, Ontario L3R 4T8.

Library of Congress Cataloging-in-Publication Data
Kirschenbaum, Daniel S., date.
The 9 truths about weight loss: the no-tricks, no-nonsense plan
for lifelong weight control / by Daniel Kirschenbaum.
p.   cm.
Includes bibliographical references and index.
ISBN 0-8050-6393-5 (hbk.)
1. Weight loss.   2. Low-fat diet.   3. Exercise.   I. Title.

RM222.2 .K546   2000   99-049927
613.7—dc21

Henry Holt books are available for special promotions
and premiums. For details contact: Director, Special Markets.

First Edition 2000

Designed by Victoria Hartman

Printed in the United States of America

1   3   5   7   9   10   8   6   4   2

Contents

Preface

According to recent bestsellers, nine truths about weight loss might be:

1. Forget about calories—fat is where it's at.
2. Forget about fat—protein is where it's at.
3. Eat equal amounts of protein and carbohydrates at every meal.
4. Stop eating potatoes, corn, rice, and sugar, and stop drinking beer.
5. Stop eating bananas, cherries, grapes, dried fruits, and pineapple. Start eating regular doses of steak and cheesecake.
6. Use an individualized diet based on your blood type.
7. Discontinue eating turkey sandwiches because they put a strain on your digestive system.
8. Arrange the food on your plate by volume so that you eat equal amounts of sloppy joe meat, asparagus with hollandaise sauce, and hot cherry cobbler à la mode.
9. Make your inner world a safe and soothing place.

The many ways that these supposed truths contradict each other show how their authors have turned science upside down looking for a new fix for this difficult problem. There are millions of overweight people who want to lose weight, but many give up before the battle is won. I hope you are among those who are truly serious about losing weight for good. Perhaps you've grown tired of quick fixes and quirky meal plans. Such approaches do not work in the long run, even though some of them may help some people in the short run. Are you ready to embrace what really works? *The 9 Truths about Weight Loss* takes a scientifically grounded and dramatic stance about how to lose weight and keep it off.

Untruths and Partial Truths for Sale

The authors of the current crop of diet books, while claiming substantial expertise, rarely have credentials directly related to weight loss. For example, very few of them have published anything at all in the professional literature about weight loss. The recycled ideas in these books reflect the pursuit of the dollar, not the offer of genuine help based on science.

Some of these books seriously distort nutritional science. Others offer "psychobabble" about the supposedly vital role that self-awareness plays in successful weight control. Weight controllers are presumed to be woefully inadequate psychologically and in dire need of self-analysis, insight, and guidance about how to resolve unconscious conflicts.

Scientific evidence indicates, however, that overweight individuals are very similar to nonoverweight individuals in overall psychological makeup and intelligence. The unconscious conflicts of overweight people, if such things even exist, probably resemble the conflicts of those who have never struggled with weight problems. Furthermore, weight-loss treatments designed to resolve such inner conflicts have failed miserably.

There are some weight-loss books that have legitimate scientific foundations. Several of these books advocate very low-fat diets. But research has demonstrated that focusing exclusively on the amount of fat eaten produces very few benefits. If you eat 3,000 calories of pasta a day, with or without fat-free tomato sauce, you will not lose weight. These books, while based on science, use science incompletely.

The most recent and successful science-based books simply do not go far enough when advocating changes in eating and exercising. For example, *Prevention's Your Perfect Weight* counsels readers to live by the motto "Everything in moderation." Unfortunately, moderation doesn't help people lose weight permanently.

Weight controllers want a long-term solution to the weight problem that plagues them every day. Pseudoscientific claims of diet breakthroughs naturally attract attention. The psychobabble solutions also maintain a certain appeal—perhaps if you gain a special type of insight, you can finally overcome the problem of excess weight. Even most of the science-based books offer the false promise that a simple idea, like very low-fat eating, can unchain the thin person within you forever.

Those who are looking for magical biological solutions, special insights, and simple solutions very understandably want to decrease the onerous qualities of the work of weight control. But for those who really want to succeed, it's time to get off the futile diet-craze treadmill and deal with the true challenges posed by excess weight. *The 9 Truths about Weight Loss* describes, in concrete terms, how to lose weight for good. Every diet-book author claims to know what works, but none has backed up each claim with real science. This book, written by an author who is both a scientist and a therapist and who has a substantial record of achievement in the field, is scientifically grounded from beginning to end. You are entitled to get the whole truth about what really works.

Advantages of the Nine Truths

The 9 Truths has three major advantages over previous weight-loss books: depth, effectiveness, and clarity. These advantages combine to make this approach a powerful prescription for lifelong change.

Depth

The 9 Truths provides a complete weight-loss program rather than the more simplistic approach of just zeroing in on very low-fat eating. *The 9 Truths* is the first book to set forth, with unassailable authority, *all* of the truths about successful weight control:

1. Your body will resist permanent weight loss.
2. Biology is not destiny.
3. Weight control is a manageable athletic challenge.
4. You will experience three stages to success: Honeymoon, Frustration, and Acceptance.
5. You can eat very little fat (20 fat grams or less) and learn how to keep your hunger quiet.
6. If you maintain a written record of your eating and exercising at least 75 percent of the time, you can manage the program successfully.
7. Exercise every day is the way.
8. You can manage stress without overeating or underexercising.
9. Maintaining weight loss is actually easier, *not* harder, than losing weight.

Effectiveness

The Nine Truths work. Nothing else really does, at least over the long haul. I have taken this position for more than twenty years in the professional literature, and many other researchers have agreed with it in recent years. My treatment program has been widely cited in such professional journals as the *American Psychologist*, *Health Psychology*, and the *International Journal of Obesity* for producing excellent results in the quest for permanent weight loss.

Consider the case of true masters of weight control. The National Weight Control Registry is a group of two thousand formerly obese people who lost an average of 60 pounds each and kept it off for an average of six years. These masters of weight control did not succeed on their first attempt. In fact, they had previously lost and regained an average of 270 pounds. A related survey found that most masters of weight control had tried to lose weight permanently at least five times before taking it off and keeping it off. When asked to compare their successes with their failures, these masters stressed that they used more intensive approaches in their successful attempts. More than 60 percent followed a much stricter dietary approach (less fat), while more than 80 percent increased their exercise.

The approach taken in *The 9 Truths* is precisely the kind of intensive approach that will help you master weight control. I personally have used this approach to lose 30 pounds and maintain that weight loss, while getting stronger and increasingly fit, for thirty years. I no longer find it particularly difficult to exercise every day (running, walking, playing tennis or golf) or to eat very little fat. Exercise makes me feel good (even youthful sometimes) and provides wonderful opportunities for me to develop friendships with some great people. I find low-fat foods, particularly spicy ethnic dishes, very enjoyable and comforting. (Yes, it's true, tasty low-fat foods can become your new "comfort foods.") I rarely feel challenged by supposedly tempting foods. Big muffins just aren't worth 50 fat grams and a slice of cheese can't justify 10 fat grams. There are other very satisfying foods readily available that won't undermine all the miles I run and the kind of life I want to lead.

You, too, can learn to master the formidable biological forces, including permanent repositories of billions of excess hungry fat cells, that resist weight loss. Those pesky fat cells never go on vacation, nor do they give partial credit for moderate, albeit sincere, effort. Tough measures are required to subdue these primitive forces. *The 9 Truths* will help you appreciate that with knowledge, commitment, and persistence, *biology is not destiny*. Thousands of my clients have mastered their biologies; athletes do this every day. You can learn to do it too!

Clarity

The 9 Truths about Weight Loss provides the clear guidelines for change that intelligent consumers want. For example, I don't just encourage you to follow conservative recommendations to eat 30 percent of your calories from fat. Better results come from a simpler goal for fat consumption: go as low as you can go. You can find creative and enjoyable ways to substitute vegetarian burgers (0 fat grams) for ground beef burgers (30 fat grams). Smother that veggie burger with honey mustard or salsa or green relish or Bermuda onions or all of that and more. Why give up eating for pleasure and comfort, like everyone else on the planet loves to do, just to avoid grease?

A New Yellow Brick Road

The 9 Truths uses the razor's edge of science to cut through the nonsense from pseudogurus. You'll learn about three stages of change that you'll experience on your journey. You'll see how and why writing down at least 75 percent of the foods you eat is necessary for success. You'll also learn why exercising every day is the way to go. It's a new road that you will see with crystal clarity. It's the same pathway that I and thousands of my clients have used to lose weight permanently. There is plenty of room on it for you.

The 9 Truths
about Weight Loss

O N E

❖

Controlling Your Body

Truth #1: Your body will resist permanent weight loss.

Truth #2: Biology is not destiny.

Truth #3: Weight control is a manageable athletic challenge.

> I eat basically the way I'm supposed to eat: rabbit food, enough
> chicken to sprout feathers, and low-fat everything. I walk more
> than most people. Yet the weight doesn't move anywhere, except
> up. I really don't get it. What else can I do?
> —Linda,* one of my frustrated clients,
> during her first session

Linda, like almost all of my clients over these past twenty-five years, didn't need me to tell her that cheeseburgers have more calories and fat than grilled chicken sandwiches. Linda worked hard to control her weight, but her approach was just not complete and intensive enough to overcome her body's resistance to weight loss.

---

*All of the case materials in this book are based directly on people whom the author has had the honor of helping during the past twenty-five years. However, the names and other aspects in each case have been changed to protect confidentiality.

Truth #1: Your body will resist permanent weight loss.

Your body's biology undoubtedly fights against weight loss every day and refuses you partial credit for sincere but moderate efforts. Linda learned to use her brain—her commitment, creativity, and persistence—to beat this biology into submission. The journey toward permanent success for weight controllers does *not* begin with the first step. It begins in earnest when all of the steps start flowing together, relentlessly tightening the noose around the neck of resistant biology. The program presented in this book will show you how to make this happen as comfortably as possible.

Beyond Moderation

Undoubtedly, the most common advice you've ever heard about losing weight is "Everything in moderation." It boils down to chicken-soup ideas like:

- "Don't try to lose weight too fast—you'll put it back on fast if you lose it too fast."
- "Don't exercise too much—you'll hurt yourself" (or "Your body needs to rest").
- "If you deprive yourself too much (especially of your favorite foods), you'll start having all-out binges."

These ideas about moderation sound plausible. Can't you just see your mother or grandmother shaking a finger at you and cajoling you about taking it easy? There's only one problem: They're wrong! Weight control doesn't follow this logical, sensible, middle-of-the-road game plan. Your biology follows its own game plan; it's a very primitive taskmaster. As Truth #1 suggests, your biology is simply too tough for such a moderate approach.

Only Highly Intensive and Consistent Efforts at Weight Control Really Work

The National Weight Control Registry includes responses to surveys by more than two thousand people who have lost, on average, 60 pounds each and kept it off for six years. These "master weight controllers" had lost, and regained, an average of 270 pounds before their successful effort took hold. Another survey of two hundred masters found that the truly successful weight-loss effort came only after an average of five previous temporarily successful weight losses. When the masters compared their successful efforts to previous attempts, the biggest difference was that they took a far more *intensive* approach. In fact, the majority of the masters used a much stricter dietary regimen (with minimal fat), and more than 80 percent reported that they exercised far more than in their previous attempts. They also reported paying far more careful attention to exactly what they ate, their weight, and their exercising during the attempts that led to long-term success. The information provided below is based on two very recent studies of highly successful weight controllers.

Masters of Weight Control: Masters of Extreme Consistency, Not Moderation

Two very recent studies by psychologists at the University of Pittsburgh and the University of Colorado provide important insights about the maintenance of weight loss. These studies involved hundreds of highly successful weight controllers and used two different samples of masters and two different types of research studies. Remarkably, the conclusions from both studies confirm the absolutely critical role of very consistent exercise, very consistent low-fat eating, and clear and frequent focusing on weight control—even many years after losing the weight initially.

One study included 714 masters who had lost, on average, 66 pounds and maintained that loss for nearly six years. The

researchers conducted an additional one-year follow-up to determine which of these masters maintained their weight (within
5 pounds of the previous year) versus those who gained at least
5 pounds.

Maintainers differed dramatically from gainers. Maintainers
weighed themselves frequently and often wrote down their eating
and exercise behaviors. They also ate very little fat and kept their
activity levels high. Gainers did not weigh themselves or record
eating and exercising data as often as the maintainers. Gainers consumed similar amounts of calories as maintainers, but gainers
increased their consumption of calories from fat by 2 percentage
points (from 23.5 percent to 25.5 percent). Note that the gainers'
level of fat consumption was still, after gaining back more than
5 pounds, much lower than the average American's (25.5 percent
versus 37 percent).

The second study gathered its participants by randomly dialing
telephone numbers across the country. The researchers found that
the 69 participants who had lost an average of 37 pounds and
maintained it for more than seven years differed, once again, in
consistency of critical weight-control behaviors compared to those
who had initially lost similar amounts of weight but regained it.
Both maintainers and gainers in this study showed substantial concern about losing weight, and much more so than a control group
that had not lost weight. Yet the maintainers differed from the
gainers in the frequency with which they weighed themselves, the
consistency of their very low-fat eating, and their high levels of
physical activity (particularly strenuous exercises). For example,
83 percent of the maintainers reported consuming less than 29
percent of their calories from fat, compared to 57 percent of the
gainers. More than 50 percent of the maintainers reported three or
more sweat-inducing physical activity episodes each week, compared to 31 percent of the gainers.

The results of these two studies show that moderation won't do
it. Only extreme levels of focus and consistency will provide the
insurance you really need, guaranteeing that the weight you lose
will stay lost.

Who are these masters of weight control? Are they obsessive freaks or only people motivated by impending and very scary medical problems? Reports in the media continually stress that less than 5 percent of weight controllers actually succeed. In 1958, physician Albert Stunkard concluded, "Most obese persons will not stay in treatment for obesity. Of those who stay in treatment, most will not lose weight, and of those who do lose weight, most will regain it." But here is the news from the late 1990s: *Modern approaches, especially those that use the extreme method set forth in this book, have produced far better results than those obtained in the first half of this century.* And you don't have to become an obsessed person on the verge of a medical disaster to lose weight. Psychologist Thomas Wadden noted recently that approximately 50 percent of people treated in the best available modern professional programs will lose 40 pounds or more, compared with only 1 percent in 1958, when Albert Stunkard reached his conclusions. That 50 percent included many perfectly reasonable, ordinary, as well as extraordinary, people.

No one who has witnessed people become masters of weight control would suggest that effective weight control is easy. It is demanding and takes genuine commitment and persistence. But thousands of people who've stayed the course have experienced radical changes in their appearance and tremendous health benefits—even reversals in serious heart disease. They have also enjoyed the elation that freedom from this dreadful problem can bring. As Sandy, one of my clients, responded when first discussing the challenges of successful weight control, "As tough as it is to lose weight and keep it off, it is much tougher to live the life of an overweight person." Sandy's success story illustrates that point.

Sandy's Success Story
236-Pound Weight Loss: "All I wanted was the truth."

Sandy was forty-two years old, five foot four, and weighed 356 pounds when she came to me four years ago. Her knees and back routinely caused her pain, and her life had become lonely and increasingly limited by her weight. Sandy never felt truly comfortable in her clothes. Everywhere she went, everyone she met, she says, "judged me by my fat first. I really hated that and almost every other part of my existence."

Sandy took to the extreme approach very eagerly. She said, "All I wanted was the truth. I learned how to make huge changes in my life and even in the way I experience emotions." For the past four years, Sandy has missed very few days of recording what she ate and totaling the number of fat grams consumed. These numbers shrank from 100 fat grams per day to the 20-grams goal suggested in *The 9 Truths*. She discovered, after some initial struggles, that "there's always something to eat that really works." She noted that only bars in Wisconsin presented nearly insurmountable problems when she was going out to eat. Most places could at least provide a piece of grilled chicken with some vegetables and/or a salad. Even when attending fixed-meal dinners, she notes, "You can usually order a vegetarian dinner that works pretty well."

Sandy began using a rowing machine that had become a haven for dust bunnies under her bed. At first she could only use it for 20 or 30 seconds at a time. She gradually increased the duration of this exercise until she could consistently work out for 30 minutes every morning before going to work. She has since added a treadmill, a big-screen TV, and a video-cassette recorder, turning her bedroom into a combination workout room and video arcade. She almost never misses a day of exercise, and she seeks out ways of staying active.

At first, all of these changes, and the consistency required for success, were quite difficult for her. Now The Nine Truths approach to weight control has become a very natural part of her life. Sandy lost 236 pounds in two years. At the time of this writing, she has maintained that weight loss for an additional two years.

The Clash of the Hunter-Gatherer Body in Twenty-first-Century Culture

You can really appreciate the importance of intensive and consistent efforts at weight control when you fully understand the biological forces within you that resist weight loss. Consider its origins in human evolution. Compare the lifestyle of our hunter-gatherer ancestors to our current culture, addicted to immediate access to information and entertainment. Imagine that you were one of our ancestors who was born in 500,000 B.C., one of the first people who had a modern human body. Consider how you would spend your days and nights when you lived with:

- No refrigerators—no means of storing food of any kind
- No weapons other than primitive spears
- No means of creating clothes other than relying on your own group's ability to skin animals and sew pieces together
- No medicine
- No means of transportation other than your feet
- No means of communication other than your voice

You and your family group would have to spend your days hunting for food, gathering food, preparing food, protecting your children, managing your primitive living conditions, creating and repairing clothes, and otherwise trying to survive, despite your physical limitations. After all, we humans don't have the strength or speed of big cats, the climbing ability and power of the great apes, or the ability to fly or to run like the wind. Our ancestors' brains and bodies had to work overtime every day to find a way to get to the next day safely.

The bodies of these early humans had to survive when the hunting yielded only exhaustion. When gathered fruits and vegetables, and perhaps insects, provided the primary foundation of our ancestors' diets, fat became a rare and precious commodity. Our bodies developed many safeguards to hang on to every bit of fat. In other words, our hunter-gatherer bodies learned how to resist weight loss aggressively so that our species, physically challenged as we were in 500,000 B.C., could survive.

Humans have lived as hunter-gatherers for 99 percent of human history. Only in the last ten thousand years did farming develop. And agricultural societies even today still suffer from food shortages every few years. A farmer's life permitted few ways to become overweight anyway, prior to the era of home deliveries and motorized dessert carts.

During the past few decades in industrial societies, our hunter-gatherer bodies began facing totally new challenges. Suddenly—very suddenly from an evolutionary perspective—some people no longer spent their days hunting and gathering or working in the fields. They began sitting around more and more. They sat down when they worked in offices; they began enjoying the luxury of sitting down for most of their days. Unfortunately, our hunter-gatherer biologies have not adapted to this luxury. Our bodies still "think" we are all hunter-gatherers, storing fat efficiently and resisting weight loss aggressively. Also, our bodies were made to move—to move a lot— for most of the day. In societies where people still move around throughout the day (China, for example), weight problems remain very rare. By contrast, our current American culture encourages very sedentary living.

It would take a major shift in environmental conditions to turn our fat-hungry biologies into fat-losing biologies. A mere hundred-year-old challenge for some of the world's population is not even a blink in time from an evolutionary perspective. As a weight con-troller, you cannot rely on your body to shift toward efficient fat burning. Our hunter-gatherer bodies will, for the foreseeable future, applaud the cookie stores on every street corner, the premium ice creams in every grocery store, and the telephones that memorize, seemingly automatically, pizza-delivery numbers. Cell phones, faxes, cable TV, DVDs, E-mail, drive-through drugstores, and other modern conveniences will continue to proliferate, making our sedentary cul-ture even more comfortable, cozy, and inactive.

Biological Barriers to Weight Control

My clients have asked me, "What exactly are these evolutionarily ordained biological forces that won't give me a break?" Let's con-sider some of the details of these biological barriers to help you appreciate and accept their power. Just remember one critical caveat as you read about them:

Truth #2: Biology is not destiny.

Each of the nine biological factors described below plays some role in making weight control quite challenging. When people develop excess weight, at any point in their lives, their bodies become espe-cially efficient and effective at maintaining higher than normal levels of fat. These biological forces include ones with which you are born, others that develop throughout your life, and still others that work to maintain high levels of body fat. Consider the power of the biology of excess weight when reviewing the nine forces described in the following sections.

It's in the Genes

Genetic factors are those that are inherited from our parents and prior generations. Mice can be selected for breeding so that fatter mice mate with other fatter mice and leaner mice with other leaner mice; over fifteen to twenty-five generations, this can produce mice pups from the fatter matings with twice as much fat as the pups from the leaner matings. This research shows the tremendous degree to which inheritance of genetic makeup determines the tendency to develop excess fat.

Human parallels include research showing that children born to parents who are both obese are four times more likely to become obese than children born to lean parents. Some recent research on twins also emphasizes the degree to which inheritance plays a role in developing excess weight. The researchers overfed twelve pairs of identical twins for one hundred days. The twins lived in a closed hospital ward and consumed about 1,000 calories per day above their normal intakes. Some pairs of twins gained more than 25 pounds during those one hundred days, whereas others who were eating the same amounts gained less than 10 pounds. If one member of a twin pair gained a lot of weight, the other member of the pair did also. In addition, the twins who gained more weight tended to gain more of the weight as fat and less of it as lean body tissues (such as muscles or organs). Other studies with twins who grew up in separate households show similar trends. They resembled each other in weight status much more than they resembled the siblings with whom they grew up. These findings make it clear that some of us are quite likely from day one to struggle with weight control, and others are more likely to be lean.

But genetics alone certainly do not determine weight. Your family and environment are also huge factors in weight control. For example, if your colleagues or friends eat high-fat lunches, that places you in a riskier environment. If your spouse exercises very regularly and loves to take walks, then at least that part of your environment supports your exercise program. It becomes obvious that environment influences weight when you look at the weight of pet owners versus their pets. Overweight people are more likely to have overweight pets than are leaner people. There is a 99.999 percent chance that humans cannot and have not mated with dogs or cats. Therefore, we share absolutely no genetic material with our pets. Yet something about the way we live affects the weight of our dogs and cats.

Fat Cells = Hungry Baby Sparrows

Beyond genetics, overweight people have many more fat cells and other biological factors that encourage them to maintain higher weights. Fat cells are like hungry baby sparrows: Both seem to open their "mouths" wider than their bodies in search of as much food as they can get. Once fat cells develop, they never disappear. Overweight people can have four times as many of these hungry creatures as their never-overweight leaner peers. People can also develop more of these insatiable beasties at any point in their lives. In fact, some research with animals shows that animals who "binge-eat" (are fed large amounts of high-fat food) can permanently gain excess fat cells within one week. Unfortunately, excess fat cells promote very efficient storage of excess food as fat.

Fat-Cell Size

Fat cells are the only ones in our bodies that can expand tremendously, seemingly at will. If you think of the smallest fat cell in the world as the size of a golf ball, then the largest fat cell would be the size of a basketball with a seven-foot diameter. That's a twenty thousand–fold difference in volume between the smallest and the largest fat cell. This tremendous elasticity allows the body to store almost unlimited amounts of fat. It seems that fat cells first increase in size as excess foods are stored in them and then they increase in number. This general tendency can change if very large amounts of food are eaten very quickly. This means that fat cells have two ways to cause problems. Either approach leads to more fat in the body and increased unhappiness.

Insulin

The concentration of blood sugar, or glucose, in our bodies is regulated very carefully in people who are not diabetic. (Diabetics are those who have major flaws in their regulation of blood sugar due to problems with the hormone insulin.) The body must maintain very careful regulation of blood sugar because the brain depends totally on blood sugar for its nutrition. If our brains aren't properly nourished, we can't survive. The body regulates the amount of blood sugar in the bloodstream by having a detector in the brain determine when blood sugar levels are too high or too low. Insulin, which is stored and manufactured in special cells within the pancreas, promotes the ingestion of glucose by our cells.

When people lose weight, the body's fat cells become especially sensitive to insulin. That enables the cells to absorb more nutrients at a faster pace. The muscle cells decrease their sensitivity to insulin, resulting in the redirection of fat to the fat cells. Several studies have shown that some people develop a greater level of insulin sensitivity when they lose weight compared to others. People who are particularly sensitive to insulin tend to regain weight very readily. It seems that a great many overweight people are quite sensitive to insulin and can very quickly store excess nutrients as fat in part because of this tendency. Most overweight people also have excessive amounts of insulin in their bloodstream at all times. This may contribute to the efficiency with which their bodies become sensitive to insulin as they lose weight.

Lipoprotein Lipase (LPL)

Lipoprotein lipase (LPL) is an enzyme (special chemical agent) produced in many cells. It stays on the walls of very small blood vessels and can become activated to transport fat in the body. During weight loss, increases in LPL in the bloodstream occur as the fat cells release their LPL into the bloodstream. By releasing LPL into the bloodstream, the fat cells send a message to the brain: "Get more food in us, now!" This means that weight loss may stimulate hunger and help convert food into stored fat. At least for some people, LPL activity seems especially high and probably makes it difficult for them to maintain weight loss.

Leptin

Leptin is another hormone that may also act as a messenger between the cells and the brain, directing the amount of fat that gets stored in fat cells. Leptin was discovered only in 1995, and it remains unclear to what extent providing additional leptin may help some people lose weight. People who show a resistance to the impact of leptin (perhaps 5 to 10 percent of overweight people) may benefit the most from ingesting more of it (if and when such a leptin drug becomes available). For most overweight people, maintaining excessive amounts of leptin in the bloodstream seems yet another mechanism to facilitate storage of fat in the fat cells.

Thermic Effect of Food

Whenever we eat something, our bodies must expend some energy to digest that food. Each type of food creates different demands for energy expenditures or thermic effects. Some research indicates that overweight people may digest their food by expending less energy (1 to 2 percent less) than never-overweight people. If your lean friend eats an apple, her body may require 10 calories beyond its normal energy demands to digest that apple. If you are an overweight person and you eat that same apple, your body may require only 9.8 calories to digest the same apple. While these tiny amounts of energy may seem trivial, they can amount to something significant over the course of days, weeks, and years. Imagine the potential benefits if it took you ten times as many calories to digest the same food as other people. This would allow you to eat many more calories while your body worked overtime to handle the food you consumed. Unfortunately, overweight people tend to be too efficient at digesting food for their own good.

Adaptive Thermogenesis

The thermic effect of food that favors lean people is part of your body's initial response when you eat something. A more long-term response is adaptive thermogenesis. When you attempt to lose weight and reduce the amount that you eat, your body has the capability of becoming very efficient. Remember the plight of the hunter-gatherers, whose bodies we share. In order for them to survive, their bodies had to make adjustments (adaptations) when they couldn't catch a deer in a particular week. Adaptive thermogenesis allowed their bodies to survive on fewer calories (greater efficiency) during times when adequate amounts of food simply weren't available. Your body can still make that quick adaptation. Instead of maintaining your weight at, say, 2,500 calories a day, when you decrease your food intake your body can maintain your weight at 1,800 calories per day. The good news about adaptive thermogenesis (which is discussed further in the chapter on exercise) is that you can reverse this effect by exercising every day. This exercise effect allows you, for example, to lose weight on 1,800 calories a day if you maintained your weight at 2,500 calories per day.

Stomach Capacity

Recent studies from Columbia University's Obesity Research Center indicate that overweight people's stomachs can hold, on average, approximately four cups of fluid. This capacity decreased by one-quarter or so when the participants in the studies lost 20 pounds. The reduction to a three-cup stomach approximates that of most people who are not overweight. Interestingly, some people who have significant problems with binge eating have stomach capacities that are especially large, even larger than that of the average overweight person.

A larger stomach probably makes it easier to eat larger meals. It also can increase hunger and appetite specifically for larger meals. The stomach seems to have special "stretching sensors" that send

signals to the brain to quiet the appetite once it is filled. The signals may not begin traveling to the brain until the stomach has almost reached its full capacity. So the more the stomach can hold, the bigger the meal needed to create a feeling of fullness.

This means that if you can decrease your weight and do it, in part, by eating smaller meals (while avoiding binges), you might decrease your stomach's capacity. This should help you feel full faster and partially tame your hungry biology. On the other hand, if you eat some big meals or binge occasionally, your stomach will stay large or get larger, making you hungry more often.

Set-Point

The notion of set-point is a way of summarizing these and other biological forces that work against long-term weight loss. As you attempt to lose weight, your body uses adaptive thermogenesis to help you become more efficient. Your body also relies on its efficient digestion of food (thermic effect) and its use of various hormones and enzymes (insulin, leptin, LPL) to make it difficult for you to lose weight and keep it off. Fat cells themselves, including their unusual ability to expand in size and number, also contribute to this problem.

The set-point is a way of summarizing all of these effects to make the point that your body will use a variety of biological forces to resist weight loss. Just as leptin has been a recent discovery, undoubtedly there are other biological mechanisms that contribute to your body's desire to maintain an excessive amount of fat. Research with animals has shown that very overweight rats and mice show similar tendencies to defend (or set) the amount of fat in their bodies at a very high level. Part of this defense (or set-point) includes a tendency for your body to respond more dramatically than people who have never had a weight problem to the sight, smell, and even the thought of tempting foods. A study by psychologists William Johnson and Hal Wildman confirmed this by showing that, compared to lean participants, overweight participants showed increased insulin responses both to the actual sight and smell of bacon and eggs, and also to the thought of bacon and eggs. This means that overweight people may defend their high weights by oversecreting insulin and digestive enzymes. This would compel them to consume more food in order to decrease the levels of these substances in the bloodstream.

Accepting the Force within You

Now it is time to accept the fact that the biology of excess weight is a real and powerful force in your life and the lives of every overweight individual. As a famous diminutive Jedi master once said, "The force is with you." There is no escaping this reality. But you can learn to manage your biological force effectively.

When I explained these biological realities to Joe, one of my clients, he became quite upset. Joe was stunned at the power of it all. He said, "I can't believe it! All of my life people, including doctors, told me that my body was basically normal, fat but normal. Now you are telling me that I am biologically abnormal and that this biology is the main cause of my weight problem? Why did I have to live the last twenty years thinking that I was so pathetic? It's not just me or my personality, right? I really have to live with something that's a physical force within me."

Joe's concerns are very legitimate. And when you think about it, the biology of obesity makes a lot of sense. Why would so many people have so much difficulty maintaining weight losses if biological forces did not oppose such weight losses? Losing weight produces many positive rewards. But relatively brief lapses in concentration (for example, binges and inconsistent exercising) are greeted eagerly by your body's extra billions of fat cells. That's a lot of hungry sparrows to feed! These fat cells and other biological forces are always present, ready to pounce.

Joe had to learn first to accept the powerful role that biology plays in creating and maintaining weight problems. Once he accepted this, he could take some of the blame away from his personality and self-esteem. Joe and the rest of us do not have to overcome our "weak" and "pathetic" personalities. We do not have to go from an abnormal state of gluttony to a normal state of controlled eating. Rather, we must change from a relatively normal state of functioning with an unfortunate biology to an extreme state. Very low-fat, low-calorie eating and very frequent exercising are necessary to overcome the biology of obesity. This makes the challenge of weight control one of the most difficult challenges a person can face.

Truth #3: Weight control is a manageable athletic challenge.

You probably know from your own experience that *diets don't work*. How many of the following have you tried?

- Special foods—provided for you at a weight-loss center
- Special foods delivered to your home
- Very low-fat diet
- High-protein and high-fat diet
- Liquid diet, milkshakes, or protein bars
- Soup, soup, soup
- Special food combinations at certain times of the day

Diets are extreme measures. Going on them does not help you create a consistent weight controller's lifestyle, which should include very low-fat eating and daily exercising. Can you learn to live that lifestyle by buying only certain prepared foods for a few weeks, by following a strange regimen of combining only certain foods together, or by focusing on pasta or on only one type of soup? You can't. Not one shred of scientific evidence shows lasting benefits from these quick fixes. Diets just don't work. They are extreme—and extremely misdirected. Serious weight controllers need serious solutions, not quick fixes and fads.

Serious athletes make very deliberate decisions about their sports. They decide to get the right equipment. They seek out qualified instructors. They decide to train at high levels to achieve their goals. Elite athletes take this several steps further than weekend warriors. They must decide to practice or train in a dedicated fashion, usually about four hours a day, nearly every day. This training helps such committed athletes overcome their resistant biologies. No one's body wants to work that hard. The body cries out to be a couch potato. The brain of these athletes must overcome this very natural biological resistance.

Clearly athletes, like weight controllers, must battle biological forces to achieve their goals. Pitting brain against biology, athletes resist rest and weight controllers resist fatty foods and sedentary living. Yet many weight controllers pursue weight loss as if they had no choice. It's as if our culture or peer or parental pressure demanded the pursuit of weight loss. But how can you rally your brain to battle your biology if you don't very actively choose to do so?

The multibillion-dollar weight-loss industry encourages you to lose weight without fully committing to this challenge. Virtually all models for goods and services seen in the media are slim. Weight-loss books and products are usually described as easy to use and guaranteed to work. If you follow this logic to its conclusion, you think:

> If you do not lose weight quickly, easily, and keep it off forever, you're either bad or dumb.

Of the many lies seen in advertising and in the public consciousness, this is one of the biggest. Overweight boys and girls experience this message and suffer for it, as do adults. Author-playwright Wendy Wasserstein poignantly describes how this message has compromised her self-esteem.

We Treat Melons Better

When I embark on any new romantic or career venture, there is for me always the same bottom line. Namely, I will assume that, no matter what happens, no matter how deeply I fall in love or how successful the project, if anything goes wrong it is because I prefer buttered rolls to bran flakes for breakfast. Or: I don't have fear of intimacy; my date has a fear of flesh.

Okay, maybe I'm exaggerating a little. But the paranoia, the impulse to blame everything on excess tonnage, is undeniably real.

More than anything it's my hope, my fantasy, that someday this horribleness will all go away. Yes, triglycerides are bad, and lack of muscle tone on someone so young is horrendous. But so is such a superficial standard for rating human quality. We treat melons with more dignity. At least we wait to make a judgment until we know what's inside.

—Wendy Wasserstein,
Bachelor Girls

Consider how athletes are treated when they do not reach their goals. Did you know that only 3 percent of professional baseball players ever play, even for one minute, in the major leagues? Are athletes condemned for failing to be the best? No! This is exactly the approach that makes the most sense for all weight controllers. When athletes shape their bodies into a supernormal condition in order to achieve supernormal feats, they receive praise and support for their efforts. When weight controllers shape their bodies into supernormal conditions via exceptional personal management skills, they deserve praise and support for their efforts too.

Essentially, *weight control is a major athletic challenge.* When you succeed as a weight controller, you deserve the same credit and admiration that we give to successful athletes. If you do not succeed, you deserve sympathy or at least acceptance. This is the best attitude to take toward yourself. If you make it and become a successful weight controller, you deserve to feel very proud of accomplishing something remarkable. If you decide not to pursue this approach, you are neither bad nor dumb. You are simply a human being exercising your right to choose how to live.

All Personal Changes Are Challenging

Weight control may pose one of the greatest lifelong personal challenges that anyone can face, but all personal changes are challenging. We all follow certain paths in our lives as a result of many very powerful influences. Your childhood, genetic makeup, early experiences, relationships with significant people, financial status, and many other factors get you walking down a certain road. Trying to get to a different pathway takes great effort and a little luck.

Consider the following research about how people resist prescribed regimens:

- *Prescriptions.* Approximately one-third of the 750 million new prescriptions written in a recent year in the United States and England were never filled. An additional 300 million of those prescriptions were not followed in the way they were written.
- *Adolescent cancer.* Approximately 50 percent of the medications prescribed to adolescents with cancer are not taken as directed.
- *Epilepsy.* Approximately 35 percent of the time, drug regimens prescribed for epilepsy are not followed.
- *Pediatric illness.* Parents fail to ensure that their children

adhere to medication regimens approximately 50 percent of the time.

- *Behavior modification for children.* Approximately 50 percent of the parents involved with behavior-modification programs for decreasing childhood problems discontinue the procedures against therapeutic advice.
- *Depression.* Approximately one-third of patients with depressive disorders discontinue their medications against medical advice.
- *Schizophrenia.* Approximately 75 percent of schizophrenic patients discontinue treatment prematurely.
- *Chronic illnesses among the elderly.* A majority of elderly people who have chronic illnesses do not follow their prescribed and necessary medication regimens.
- *Kidney disease.* Approximately 70 percent of patients with kidney disease fail to follow dietary and fluid restrictions necessary for their comfort and health.
- *High blood pressure.* Only 30 percent of people with high blood pressure follow the medical regimens that can save their lives.
- *Exercise.* Only 20 percent of adult Americans exercise at least twice a week for at least 30 minutes. The American College of Sports Medicine recommends that everyone should exercise at least four times per week.
- *Diabetes.* Only about 7 percent of diabetic patients adhere to all of the steps considered necessary for good control of this deadly disease.

These statistics startle some people. I've heard questions like, "How can people fail to take medications and follow other steps that are so critical to preserving their health and well being?" In some ways, this perfectly reasonable question misses the point. The fact is that people usually have to struggle to maintain regimens of any kind that are different from what they are used to doing. Almost regardless of the consequences, we resist change mightily.

In their book *Facilitating Treatment Adherence*, psychologists Donald Meichenbaum and Dennis Turk offer a remarkable example of how people resist change despite sometimes dire consequences. They describe a study by Patricia Vincent on glaucoma, a serious but treatable eye disease. Patients who were diagnosed with glaucoma were told that they must use eye drops three times per day or *they would go blind*. Vincent reported that only 42 percent of these patients used the eye drops frequently enough to avoid permanent damage to their vision. Only 28 percent of the people who had not adhered to the regimen improved their use of the eye drops even after they reached the point of becoming legally blind in one eye!

These statistics also raise an important point about weight control. Since most people struggle in any attempt to change their lifestyles, why are overweight people criticized so harshly for having this problem? Consider the blame factor. Children as well as adults *blame* overweight individuals for their excess weight. If someone is an epileptic or diabetic, they are regarded as blameless and unfortunate. But people do not believe the first and most basic truth about losing weight. They just don't believe that biological forces make weight control very challenging. They see excess weight as a product of gluttony and personal inadequacy. The thinking is, "If you are overweight, you must eat too much and you must be too lazy or too weak to change."

Remember that persistence toward intensity and consistency makes change possible. Athletes can become highly skilled; most diabetics can control all aspects of their disease effectively; people with high blood pressure can control it; and overweight people can use the steps I've outlined to lose weight permanently. You can learn how to stay in the struggle even when your scale betrays

you. None of these things are easy, but all of them are possible—
with commitment, knowledge of the Nine Truths, and persistence.

> Extremism in pursuit of permanent lifestyle change is no vice.
> Moderation in defense of failure to change is no virtue.

T W O

❖

Stages of Change

I think I can. I think I can. I think I can. . . . *I can!*

versus

I think I can't. I think I can't. I think I can't. . . . *I can't!*

Truth #4: You will experience three stages to success: Honeymoon, Frustration, and Acceptance.

Great (and Not So Great) Expectations

If you expect to succeed, you really might; if you expect to fail, you probably won't succeed. These assertions are surprisingly accurate. Psychologists have studied the power of positive thinking for more than sixty years, and while it alone cannot get you to walk an hour a day or order fruit instead of cheesecake, believing in the possibility of positive change works much better than pessimism.

The following examples illustrate that improving expectations can change pain to pleasure, increase motivation, and perhaps decrease illness. As you read these, consider the benefits of improving your expectations for long-term success in weight control.

Mind over Taco

Psychologist Irving Kirsch relates the following story: I always liked Mexican food, but I didn't like hot spicy food; in fact, I found the experience painful. Even a radish made me feel uncomfortable. I coped with this dilemma by frequenting Tex-Mex restaurants only in the gringo neighborhoods of Los Angeles, ordering just the safe foods—burritos, tostados, cheese enchiladas, and frijoles. The hot sauce sat safely at the end of the table, untouched.

[A few remarkable things changed my interest in spicy foods forever during a recent trip to a local Mexican eatery. I realized that] when you take your first bite of a hot dish, there is a short period of time during which you can taste the flavor of the food, before it is eclipsed by the fiery sensation of the spice. During that brief delay, the delicious flavor of the guacamole taco came through. But then came the pain—excruciating pain! A familiar searing sensation spread through my mouth, and my eyes began to water.

Normally at that point, I would swallow the offending substance as quickly as possible and grope for a glass of water. But that afternoon, I did not. A sudden insight had occurred to me. Recalling the marvelous flavor that the pain had obscured, and seeing the expressions of pleasure on the faces of my friends, I thought: "Why am I experiencing pain while they are experiencing pleasure? The tacos are the same, and there is nothing physically different between them and me. We have the same kinds of taste buds, the same type of pain receptors. It's not fair! I too should be able to enjoy a guacamole taco."

I decided to try to experience exactly what my friends were experiencing by changing my expectations from "pain" to "pleasure." So I did not swallow as quickly, nor did I reach for a glass of water. Instead, I chewed slowly. I rolled the food around in my mouth. I savored it. The taco still tasted spicy, but the spiciness was no longer painful. It began to feel pleasant, and finally, wonderful.

From that day on, my experience of spicy food has been different; it is no longer painful. When it is good and spicy, it is spicy and good.

Mind over Muscle

Twenty-four men were tested for arm strength. Subjects were then paired and asked to arm wrestle each other. The researchers arranged the pairs so that one man was clearly stronger than the other. Incorrect information was provided to both wrestlers, so that both opponents expected the objectively weaker man to win. In other words, before actually wrestling, both men believed that the stronger man was actually the weaker man. Ten of the twelve contests (83 percent) were won by the man who had tested weaker! These results suggest that expectations can overcome physical strength.

Mind over Poison Ivy

Thirteen boys were touched on their left arms with leaves that looked like poison ivy. These leaves were harmless, but the boys were told that the leaves sometimes caused irritations to the skin. They were touched on their right arms with leaves that they believed were harmless. Actually, these leaves were from a plant that creates a skin rash similar to poison ivy (from a lacquer, or "wax," tree). "Reality" suggests that none of the boys should have developed any skin reactions on their left arms and that all of them should have had reactions on their right arms (based on the actual qualities of the leaves themselves). Amazingly, all thirteen boys developed a skin reaction to the harmless leaves (on their left arms), while only two reacted to the leaves from the lacquer tree on their right arms. Here again, expectations overcame "reality."

Expectations and Losing Weight: "I THINK I CAN"

These examples of the power of expectations apply directly to weight control. What do you expect right now from your efforts at weight control? Are your expectations more like Jane's or Barbara's?

> *Jane:* "I really can't imagine living my life on a diet. I think people have to experiment with their eating. I just need to eat

burgers and french fries sometimes. I also can't imagine exercising every day or even almost every day. What if I just don't feel like exercising sometimes? I'm not sure if I'm ready to live my life like a nun."

Barbara: "I would love to learn how to actually enjoy exercising. I have never exercised consistently. I think I can learn to focus on exercising and find a way to make exercising a part of my life. There are times when I actually seem to prefer eating in the right way, as well. I am hoping and expecting that I can make low-fat eating a part of my daily routine. I don't want to keep fighting it anymore."

If your expectations are more like Jane's than Barbara's, you have a lot of work to do. Jane expects to struggle and seems to resent the process. Barbara expects to change and almost looks forward to the process. Perhaps it would make sense for Jane to talk with people who have become effective weight controllers. She would find that many of them take pride in their abilities to control their eating and exercising. Successful weight controllers also feel good after exercising. Even people who have not overcome weight problems learn to enjoy the way it feels to exercise and the health benefits exercising brings. If Jane talks with committed exercisers and successful weight controllers, she may start to believe she can succeed.

Stages of Change

What would happen if you expected to lose 100 pounds in one year and you lost only 30? What would happen if you expected to remain optimistic and positive when pursuing effective weight control and you found yourself becoming annoyed and frustrated instead? The road to successful weight control is bumpy, so it helps to understand and anticipate the nature of the bumps and how to cope with them. Developing a good understanding of what to expect can improve your commitment and help you appreciate the benefits of extreme weight control.

Weight controllers experience certain phases or stages along the way to successful persistence. The illustration below shows the three primary stages of change. Each stage consists of characteristic, or typical, behaviors, thoughts, and feelings. That is, people in each stage tend to act and think in similar ways. Most people experience all three stages during their first two years of committed effort at weight control. By considering the nature of each stage you may improve your expectations for success.

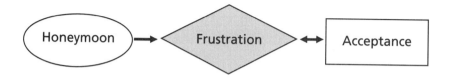

Fig. 2.1
Stages of Change in Successful Weight Control

Honeymoon

Thoughts and feelings. Weight controllers in this stage often express delight and a sense of genuine satisfaction. They seem relieved and eager to take control of this difficult problem.

Behaviors. Honeymooners consistently attend weight-control sessions if they're participating in a formal program. They also carefully observe themselves by keeping records of their eating and exercising. They read about weight control and exercise, and they also talk with other people about health, weight control, and related topics. In other words, honeymooners rather eagerly practice extreme weight control.

Example. Lisa was a thirty-five-year-old nurse who was married and had two young children when I first met her. She had a busy and very fulfilling life. Unfortunately, she had gained 50 pounds over the last five years after she quit smoking and had two children. Even before, Lisa's weight was more than she wanted it to be—just on the high side of the normal range. She described much of her eating as "something to soothe me. It helped me feel calmer—at least for a little while." Eating ice cream and cookies became a means of coping.

Lisa began participating in a therapy group that I conducted. She was annoyed, angry, depressed, and eager to change. She grabbed onto the ideas and principles that we discussed in the group and kept meticulous records of what she ate and when she exercised. Lisa was pursuing persistence at weight control. She was "going for it"! She seemed very committed, dedicated, and happy to have a chance to tame this difficult problem.

Lisa's monitoring of her eating and exercising remained meticulous and complete for about twelve months. She did not resent the effort required for her to achieve a 30-pound weight loss during that year. She showed remarkable enthusiasm and concentration. Weight loss became a focal point for her. Lisa's attitude and efforts also helped encourage and inspire the rest of the group members.

Frustration

Thoughts and feelings. In this stage, people often think about going back to their old ways of eating and exercising. They seem to long for the old days. After all, the old ways are easier and take much less time and energy. People in the Frustration stage resent the effort required for successful weight control. They compare themselves to people who are not overweight and those who have never been overweight. This is a "Why me?" stage. "Why do I have to work at this all the time?" "Why can't I take a break from the effort every once in a while?" "Why doesn't my spouse have to suffer with this biology?" In this stage, weight controllers battle life's basic unfairness.

Behaviors. Weight controllers in this stage become less careful about their eating and exercising, not monitoring as well as in the Honeymoon stage. If they are attending a formal program, they may have more difficulties getting to the meetings and arriving on time. The expression "hanging in there" (sometimes just barely) describes this well.

Example. Lisa eventually reached the Frustration stage. After a year of hard work, dedication, and effectiveness at weight control, she began struggling. During this stage, she talked about resenting how easy it was for her husband to "eat whatever he wants." Her rate of weight loss slowed, and it became more difficult for her to keep accurate records of her eating and exercising. She refused to give up, but her feelings changed from eagerness to frustration. "Why me?" was a consistent theme in Lisa's comments in the group. She could not understand or accept her rate of weight loss either. The year before, if she didn't lose weight during one particular week, she would say, "No problem. It'll happen. I'm on track." In this stage, she said, "I can't believe this! I'm eating practically nothing and look what happens! Nothing!"

Acceptance

Thoughts and feelings. This is a stage in which people settle in for the long haul. They experience *a peaceful sense of resolve* about weight control. They feel comfortable, with a clear direction for handling their challenging biologies. They also refine their knowledge of nutrition in this stage, and their understanding of the factors that affect weight control becomes clearer as well. They still struggle with their focusing or commitment, however. This happens quite often when they go on vacations or when their schedules are disrupted by illness or travel.

Behaviors. When weight controllers reach the Acceptance stage, they have developed very consistent patterns of exercise. They view exercise as either enjoyable or at least acceptable, no longer seeing it as drudgery but as something that can help them. So they maintain more positive and effective attitudes toward it.

In this stage, weight controllers consistently monitor their food and exercise. They also assert themselves effectively in restaurants and other social situations regarding food. For example, weight controllers in this stage would not accept a meal they had ordered "grilled, as dry as possible" if it was served swimming in butter. They would ask their server to have the fish or chicken prepared again. Weight controllers in the Acceptance stage do not battle themselves anymore about ordering low-fat, low-calorie meals, nor do they feel deprived and frustrated when they ask for their food to be prepared in a healthful way. They feel taken care of and happier when they can get food prepared the way they now "prefer." I put the word "prefer" in quotes very deliberately. Can you really prefer baked potatoes to french fries? Fresh berries to chocolate mousse? Cheese-less pizza to sausage or pepperoni (and cheese, of course) pizza? "No way!" one of my clients replied when asked that question. "I'll eat the healthier alternatives, but no one can convince me that low fat tastes better than high fat. Be real!"

Weight controllers in this stage still sometimes struggle with certain situations and still experience eating and exercising lapses (even binges occasionally). Just as disruptions in routines (vacations, travel) alter commitment or focus, these kinds of disruptions change behaviors too. Travel and vacations change routines and rules. Snacking during the day, for example, may not occur during a typical work week. During vacations, on the other hand, the opportunities to snack increase, and the "I deserve it" rationales re-emerge.

Example. Lisa did come out of the Frustration stage and went into the Acceptance stage, having begun to realize that her frustration was getting her nowhere. Sure, her biology was much more difficult to manage than her husband's and other more fortunate people around her. Who said life was fair? She saw the challenge before her as something that she could accomplish. She realized that she had maintained a substantial weight loss. Even if she never lost another pound, she noted, at least she wasn't gaining weight anymore. She could now fit into many more of her clothes, and she felt better about herself. Lisa's feelings shifted from frustration and anger to a calmer, more peaceful state. She still had trouble sometimes with vacations and other major disruptions in her routines. During these times she occasionally developed a "vacation mentality," and this "give myself a break" attitude led to more problematic eating. She learned to recover from these lapses very effectively, however. She restarted her monitoring of eating and exercising as soon as she got home and reinforced her own refusal to give up. She could even laugh about her vacation mentality. She realized that her fat cells took no vacations. They remained ever eager to pounce on those extra calories. They loved her vacations!

Evaluating Your Own Stage of Change

Which stage of change are you currently experiencing? To answer this critical question, let's consider several additional profiles. The examples below tell us about three individuals, Michael, Susan, and Janet. Take a look at their case histories and note how people move through the stages of change. See if you can use their examples to help you identify your current stage of change.

Three Examples of Moving through the Stages of Change

· ·

Michael: Honeymoon to Frustration

Michael was incredibly eager to embrace all of the ideas presented in his professionally conducted program, which was designed to help people improve their abilities to focus and modify their eating and exercising habits. He was a very attentive group member, and he also completed every possible task presented to him on time and in great detail. His recording of his eating was impeccable. Michael gradually increased his daily exercising from a 5- to 10-minute walk to a 45-minute fast walk. He lost 1 to 3 pounds almost every week.

Quite unexpectedly, during his third month of the program, Michael began missing group sessions. His eating records became spotty, and he began complaining about the demands of the program. He reported substantial binges that occurred several times per week. Michael discontinued his involvement in the program and did not answer either telephone or written correspondence from his group leader.

Susan: Honeymoon to Frustration to Acceptance

Susan also participated in a professional weight-control program. She was approximately 120 pounds overweight but was eager to change. She began exercising by walking and occasionally swimming. As she became more fit, she bought a treadmill for her use at home. She eventually joined a health club and began lifting weights and stretching with the help of a professional trainer. Her exercising was very consistent and quite extensive. Susan reported great joy in her exercising and in the challenge of weight lifting. She followed a very low-calorie regimen (approximately 800 calories per day), relying on frozen dinner entrées for most of her lunch and dinner meals. This helped her keep the calorie levels well controlled. She avoided restaurants and parties and lost weight rapidly. She reported that it seemed "easy" for the first eleven months of her program.

In her twelfth month, Susan suffered a back injury during one of her workouts, and this was quickly followed by a serious bout with the flu. These setbacks seemed to derail her. Her exercising was slowed down considerably due to the injury and illness. She attempted to re-engage exercising as quickly as possible but had to yield to her physical limitations. Her eating began to include binges on cookies and other foods that are high in fat and sugar. Her monitoring changed from perfectly consistent to quite inconsistent, and she reported great annoyance at the unfairness of her physical maladies.

In her twenty-first month, Susan finally decided that this was one aspect of her life that she could control. She reinitiated her monitoring on a consistent basis. Her exercising did not go back to the level it had been during her first year, but she became more consistent, and she varied her exercising to accommodate her back injury. Susan talked about feeling more committed and more willing to face the problem of her binge eating head-on.

Janet: Frustration to Honeymoon to Frustration

Janet had difficulty monitoring. She understood the rationale for it completely, but she "didn't want to face it." Janet avoided talking in her Take Off Pounds Sensibly (TOPS) group. Other TOPS members tried to encourage her to discuss her feelings. Janet resisted. She sometimes arrived at her group late and seemed to fidget or read. She didn't seem to want to be there.

Janet gradually began talking more in the group. Her discussions included emphasizing why weight control was important to her. Her monitoring improved dramatically. She began losing weight consistently.

In her tenth month, Janet took a vacation to Europe. Upon returning, she reported to her group that she had "lost her focus completely." She talked about being around other people who didn't have to worry about this problem. She had trouble facing the nature of her biology and the inherent unfairness of it. Her attendance was consistent, but her efforts were not.

Michael, Susan, and Janet experienced weight control in different ways during their efforts to change. Michael began the program with great enthusiasm that landed him solidly in the Honeymoon stage. However, by the third week he became lost in the Frustration stage and relatively quickly disengaged from the entire process. Susan's Honeymoon stage lasted almost a full year. An injury threw her into the Frustration stage. However, she was able to rebound from this challenging time and get herself into the Acceptance stage around the time of the second anniversary of this major effort at weight control. Janet never seemed to experience a Honeymoon stage at all. Or you might decide that she experienced a delayed Honeymoon stage that began after an early Frustration stage. Her initial ambivalence to the process of losing weight resurfaced after about ten months, and she had a major disruption in her routine (a vacation to Europe), after which she became entrenched, once again, in a Frustration stage.

Toward Successful Weight Control through the Stages of Change

No one learns to master weight control in a straight line. Like Michael, Susan, and Janet, you will experience bumps in the road toward success. You may get into a Honeymoon stage that lasts several weeks, several months, or even a year. During that wonderful time, the process may seem relatively easy. But, as in the cases of Michael, Susan, and Janet, experiencing the Frustration stage is virtually inevitable. The difference between Michael's efforts at weight control versus Susan's and Janet's has to do with persistence. Michael ran into the wall of Frustration and backed off completely from what he had been attempting to do so diligently for several months. In contrast, Susan and Janet maintained their involvement in their efforts and found a way to get through difficult Frustration stages. Getting through Frustration often involves continuing to participate in a structured program of some kind, despite relatively poor progress or some major change in motivation. It also involves continuing to exercise even though the scale does not reflect that kind of effort. In other words, if you find a way to maintain your habits and your focus and you absolutely refuse to give up on yourself, you can get through even the most difficult Frustration stage.

On the other side of Frustration you can find Acceptance. Ideally, as you become firmly committed to Acceptance, you will develop an attitude of *aggressive self-protectiveness*. That means you will maintain your focus despite distractions of settings, situations, or time. If you have this level of Acceptance, you can go on vacations or go over to someone else's house for dinner and handle whatever challenges come your way. You essentially have a *peaceful sense of resolve* about your body and what it requires to succeed in this incredibly challenging task. As John, one of my clients, explained, "It's my body; that's the way it works." As John felt, and hundreds of my clients have experienced over the years, why rail against your own biology? If you can find a way of accepting it and living with it, you can take charge of it. After all, many people face many other more difficult and unpleasant aspects of living. Weight control does not place you in a jail cell and demand that you only eat water and gruel. You have a wide range of foods to choose from. Many of the foods can be quite satisfying and comforting. Why not just accept your particular range of food for what it is, learn to enjoy it, and fully embrace the challenges of successful weight control?

The Power of Positive Expectations

Before 1900, patients who sought medical treatment were "purged, puked, poisoned, punctured, cut, cupped, blistered, bled, leeched, heated, frozen, sweated, and shocked," according to Arthur Shapiro's 1978 article in the *Handbook of Psychotherapy and Behavior Change*. Irving Kirsch, in his 1990 book *Changing Expectations*, noted that the "medications" prescribed by the physician in the nineteenth century and earlier included lizard's blood, crocodile dung, pig's teeth, putrid meat, fly specks, frog's sperm, powdered stone, human sweat, worms, spiders, furs, and feathers. These "treatments" have been shown to have no physical properties that could lead to a cure of anything. In fact, some of them could certainly cause harm. Yet, amazingly, some people felt better after such bizarre ministrations! Our great-great-grandparents must have *believed* in these treatments. Modern medicine still relies on the power of such positive expectations. The medicine of yesteryear relied almost exclusively on this power. Consider what you can do if you harness this force for weight control.

THREE

❖

Quieting Your Hunger

Truth #5: You can eat very little fat (20 fat grams or less) and learn how to keep your hunger quiet.

This chapter can help you tame those savage little beasts, those extra 10 or 50 billion fat cells, that make their presence known to your appetite. Thousands of very successful weight controllers have managed to tame these hungry sparrow-beasts; you can too.

In this chapter you will learn that two things have the greatest effects on your hunger: the fat content and the sugar content of what you eat. You will also learn about the ten principles of the "Almost Never" eating plan. You will find the principles of the Almost Never Eating Plan far more sensible, but more challenging, than the entirely fallacious Top Ten Rules for Easier Weight Control in a Saner, Fairer World.

Top Ten Rules for Easier Weight Control in a Saner, Fairer World

10. Food consumed for medicinal purposes doesn't have any calories. This includes throat lozenges, cough drops, chicken noodle soup, and anything bought in a Jewish deli.

9. Using sugar substitutes in coffee entitles you to a free dessert every once in a while. Every once in a while includes two Fridays on either side of your birthday and every Saturday night, except for the second Saturday in February.

8. Snacks consumed after midnight don't count because "it could have been a dream, anyway."

7. Pieces of cookies, bagels, and cheese (not cubes or slices) have no calories. The process of breaking uses more calories than the pieces contain.

6. If you drink a diet soda with pretzels or popcorn, the pretzels and popcorn have no calories. First of all, the pretzels and (low-fat) popcorn are healthy snacks, anyway. Second, the calories in these good snacks are canceled by the diet soda.

5. If you eat with someone else, the calories you consume don't count if you eat less than they do.

4. Foods that have the same color have the same number of calories—for example, tomato sauce and cherry pie, yogurt and cheesecake.

3. Tasting food while preparing it is not really eating. Licking peanut butter off the knife while making a sandwich for your son or daughter is necessary to ensure the adequacy of the peanut butter and, therefore, no calories are consumed during this important parental task.

2. If you eat something very quickly and/or if no one sees you eat it, it has no calories. Maybe it never happened?

1. Snacks eaten at movies or theaters (for example, Milk Duds, buttered popcorn, Tootsie Rolls, chocolate Bon Bons) have no calories because they are part of the entire entertainment experience.

Good-bye Fat

The weight-control plan that I recommend focuses on managing fat and sugar in your life. This plan works best when your overall style of eating is grounded in a healthful approach to food. The Healthy-Eating Basics described below provide the key to helping you

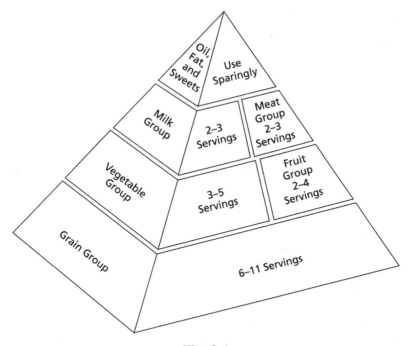

Fig. 3.1
The Food Guide Pyramid

develop a balanced, healthful foundation for your weight-control efforts.

Healthy-Eating Basics: The Food Guide Pyramid

To encourage Americans to eat a varied and balanced diet, and thereby consume adequate amounts of vitamins, minerals, and fiber, the U.S. Department of Agriculture officially launched the Food Guide Pyramid in 1992. The pyramid, shown above, presents five food groups, with the grain group (bread, cereal, rice, and pasta) at the base, illustrating that these complex carbohydrates are the foundation of a healthy diet.

As you can see, the Department of Agriculture (and the American Dietetic Association) recommends six to eleven servings per day from the grain group; two to four servings per day from the fruit group; three to five servings per day from the vegetable group; two to three servings per day from the meat group; and two to three servings per day from the milk group. The tip of the pyramid is an "others" category, for foods that do not have enough nutrients to fit into any of the five major food groups. These foods include fats and oils, sweets, salty snacks, alcohol, soft drinks, and condiments. Certainly for the fats, oils, and sweets group, weight controllers do better when they minimize consumption of these foods.

Following are descriptions of the contents of a serving for each of the five food groups with some examples of recommended foods for each.

Milk Group: Two to Three Servings. One serving equals 1 cup of milk or yogurt, 1½ ounces of natural cheese, or 2 ounces of processed cheese. Good examples are:

- Skim and 1 percent low-fat milk
- Buttermilk made with skim or 1 percent low-fat milk
- Yogurt made with skim or 1 percent low-fat milk
- Low-fat or dry-curd cottage cheese (1 to 2 percent)
- Cheeses with 2 or fewer grams of fat per ounce
- Frozen dairy desserts with 2 grams of fat or less per item or per ½ cup serving

Meat Group: Two to Three Servings. One serving equals 2 to 3 ounces of cooked lean meat, fish, or poultry; 1 to 1½ cups of cooked dried beans; 2 to 3 eggs; or 4 tablespoons of peanut butter. Good examples are:

- Beef: eye of round, top round, low-fat beef products
- Veal: all cuts except loin, rib, and ground
- Chicken or turkey without skin
- Poultry cold cuts with up to 1 gram of fat per ounce
- All fresh fish and shellfish; canned fish, water-packed, drained

- All dried beans, peas, and lentils
- Egg whites and low-fat egg substitutes

Vegetable Group: Three to Five Servings. One serving equals 1 cup of raw, leafy vegetables; ½ cup of other vegetables (cooked or chopped raw); or ¾ cup of vegetable juice. Good examples are:

- All fresh vegetables or frozen vegetables without sauce
- Canned vegetables
- Vegetable juices

Fruit Group: Two to Four Servings. One serving equals 1 medium apple, banana, or orange; ½ cup of chopped, cooked, or canned fruit; or ¾ cup of fruit juice. Good examples are:

- All fresh fruit (except avocados and olives)
- Unsweetened applesauce
- Dried fruit
- Canned fruit in its own juice

Grain Group: Six to Eleven Servings. One serving equals 1 slice of bread; 1 ounce of ready-to-eat cereal; or ½ cup of cooked cereal, rice, or pasta. Good examples are:

- Bread, bagels, pita, English muffins, rolls with 2 or fewer grams of fat
- Air-popped popcorn, pretzels, rice cakes, bread sticks, corn tortillas
- Crackers with 1 gram or less of fat per ½ ounce: melba toast, matzo, flat bread, saltines
- Cold cereals with 2 or fewer grams of fat and 6 or fewer grams of sugar per serving (for example, Cheerios, Shredded Wheat, Grape-Nuts)

- Hot cereals
- Rice, barley, bulgur wheat, couscous, kasha
- Pasta
- Low-fat pancakes and waffles

If your eating plan follows the guidelines provided by the Food Guide Pyramid, you probably will not benefit from taking vitamin or mineral supplements of any kind. You can also see by the examples that many low-fat, low-calorie foods can be used to create a balanced meal plan.

Fat Begets Fat

"Any pig farmer knows that you can't get pigs fat feeding them wheat; you need corn, which contains more oil," says Professor Elliot Danforth. Danforth and his colleague Ethan Sims, both professors at the University of Vermont, studied the causes of obesity. Using male prisoners as subjects, they asked the men to eat large amounts of food and then observed the effects. They found that the prisoners who ate a lot of high-fat foods gained much more weight than those who ate foods that were lower in fat and higher in carbohydrates.

More recent studies also show that high-fat foods are most easily stored as additional fat in the body. For example, to turn 100 calories of very high-fat food like butter or bacon into body fat, your body only expends about 3 calories of energy. That means that 97 of the 100 calories end up in your fat cells. Turning carbohydrates into fat is much more complicated. The body has to change the carbohydrate into a number of other chemical compounds in order to process it. As a result, in order to turn 100 calories of spaghetti into fat, the body has to expend about 23 calories. In other words, it costs very little energy to transform foods that already start out as fat into body fat. Therefore, 100 calories of spaghetti may translate into 77 calories of fat, whereas 100 calories of butter transform into 97 calories of fat.

Your biology (assuming you are overweight) makes it especially easy for you to gain weight. Why make a bad situation worse by eating fat?

Fat Goal: How Low Can You Go?

In order to avoid eating fat, you need to know how to measure the amount of fat in your diet. One way to calculate the fat is to determine the percentage of the total calories you consume that come from fat. Although certain types (like saturated fats) create more health problems than other types of fat (for example, monounsaturated fats, such as olive oil and peanut oil), from a weight-control perspective, *a fat is a fat is a fat*. In other words, all fats contain approximately the same number of calories. And all fats are stored by your body as fat very readily. In this respect:

> 1 tablespoon of peanut oil = lard = corn oil = coconut oil = butter = *120 calories* and *13.6 fat grams*.

So the question of greatest concern to those who want to lose weight is, "How much fat am I eating?" not "What kind of fat am I eating?"

To calculate the percentage of your calories that come from fat, first you must know the total number of calories you consume for a particular day. Then you will want to determine the number of fat grams you consumed. Since each gram of fat contains 9 calories, you can use simple arithmetic to translate the number of fat grams eaten per day to the percentage of calories consumed that day from fat. Consider the examples presented here:

CHICKEN SANDWICH

Ingredients	Calories	Fat Grams
Chicken (3 ounces)	142	3
Light wheat bread (2 slices)	80	1

Ingredients	Calories	Fat Grams
Lettuce (1 leaf)	3	0
Tomato (2 slices)	12	0
Mustard or no-fat mayonnaise (1 teaspoon)	8	0
Apple (1 medium)	80	1
Diet Coke or iced tea	0	0
Total calories	325	
Total fat grams		5

Number of fat grams × number of calories per gram (9) = calories from fat: $5 \times 9 = 45$

Percent of calories consumed from fat = calories from fat divided by total calories: $45 \div 325 = 14\%$

MCDONALD'S BIG MAC MEAL

	Calories	Fat Grams
McDonald's Big Mac	572	34
McDonald's fries (small)	222	12
McDonald's chocolate shake	356	10
Total calories	1,150	
Total fat grams		56

Number of fat grams × number of calories per gram (9) = calories from fat: $56 \times 9 = 504$

Percent of calories consumed from fat = calories from fat divided by total calories: $504 \div 1,150 = 44\%$

The McDonald's Big Mac Meal certainly outweighs the chicken sandwich meal in all ways. It includes approximately four times as many calories and eleven times as much fat as the chicken sandwich meal. These examples show more than the obvious differences between these choices for lunch. Very few weight controllers choose McDonald's Big Mac meals as the mainstay of their diets. However, this meal, as well as the chicken sandwich meal, illustrate that measuring the amount of fat in your diet requires attention to the number of fat grams consumed and the total number of calories consumed.

Specific Fat Goal: 20 Fat Grams (or Fewer) per Day

Some recent studies indicate that obese people tend to get higher percentages of their calories from fat than lean people do. Some obese people eat similar numbers of total calories compared to nonobese individuals, but the percentages of fat in their diets can be 25 percent higher. If you want to lose weight, you must consume very low percentages of fat every day. The American Heart Association suggests that if Americans adopted a diet consisting of 30 percent of calories from fat, there would be much less heart disease in this country. Right now Americans consume closer to 36 percent of their total calories from fat. Reducing to diets containing 30 percent fat would surely improve the health of many people; but this level is still too high for people who wish to lose weight. Most experts recommend that a better percentage for weight controllers is 20 percent. My recommendation is even simpler than that: Consume as low a percentage of your total intake from fat as you can tolerate. So the answer to the question, "How low can you go?" is: "As low as possible!" For most people, this means aiming for *20 fat grams* per day or less.

Living with a very low-fat eating plan presents many challenges. This is the age of motorized dessert carts and specialty cookie shops on every street corner. While people talk about exercising more than ever before, many people exercise as a way of justifying high-fat eating. Who can forget the image of President Bill Clinton jogging to a fast-food restaurant? Others enjoy wearing exercise clothes; but participating is a different story. The same applies to living life without high-fat foods. For example, in a recent *Consumer Reports* article entitled "Are You Eating Right?" the editors noted that Americans were "still saying 'cheese.'" That is, "Americans have soured on whole milk in the past 25 years and now choose low-fat milk more often. But consumption of high-fat cheeses has more than doubled in the same period, and even cream is rising."

All successful weight controllers consume much less fat in their eating plans than do average Americans. This means that they rarely eat red meat, hardly ever eat desserts other than fruit or low-fat or no-fat alternatives, and almost never eat fried foods. Their salad dressings are almost always fat-free, low-fat, or low-calorie, and when they order salads in restaurants, they order the salad dressings on the side. They grill and broil and bake and steam foods, and they insist on being served foods prepared in those low-fat ways in restaurants. Successful weight controllers rarely eat anything with gravy or sauces (other than broths and simple tomato sauces). No-fat or low-fat cheeses, ice cream, and mayonnaises are also among their possibilities. They think of normal-fat cookies, brownies, cake, and candy as foods for others, not for themselves.

Many people really *can* live this way. For example, if you have made the change from whole milk to skim milk, do you miss drinking whole milk, or does it seem more like cream to you now? People find some of these changes easier to implement than you might expect. For example, consider the following comments from some of my more successful clients:

- "It's amazing, but I don't even want candy anymore. When I see candy, or people eating candy, I don't have the slightest interest in eating it."
- "I find fried foods disgustingly greasy now. Except for french fries, fried foods don't tempt me in the least. Okay, maybe onion rings tempt me a little too."
- "This is the best time in history for living with fat-free and low-fat foods. There are so many perfectly good choices."
- "I now think of high fat-foods as 'alien foods.' I say to myself, 'That stuff is for people from other worlds.' "

Low-Fat Eating Tips

Some ideas about foods that have helped my clients make low-fat eating more palatable include:

- Snacks: air-popped popcorn, pretzels, fruit, rice cakes, sugar-free Jell-O, low-calorie cocoa, the usual raw vegetables (pre-peeled minicarrots are especially good).
- Mustard on everything; collect, compare, and contrast many different varieties of mustards.
- Learn to love spicy foods.
- Salsa on everything: Become a salsa connoisseur and collect, compare, and contrast many different varieties.
- Pasta, pasta, pasta.
- Tomato sauces, particularly low-fat versions.
- Fish, shellfish.
- Stir-fried cooking: Use broths, water, no oil if possible.
- No-fat cheeses: Try melting them on bagels or English muffins.
- Baked potatoes with dry, 1 percent cottage cheese or very low-fat yogurt instead of sour cream. Did you know that a baked medium sweet potato has 100 calories less than a medium baked white potato (118 versus 220)?
- Soups: Experiment with vegetables, beans, bones.
- Frozen entrées that specify amount and percent of fat (limit your choices to those with no more than 20 percent of total calories from fat). Examples with 10 percent of calories from fat or less: Healthy Choice ravioli, Healthy Choice linguini with shrimp, Tyson roasted chicken, and Ultra Slim-Fast mesquite chicken.
- Canned no-fat soups.
- Use applesauce or the new oil- and shortening-replacement products made from fruit purees instead of butter and oil in baked goods.
- When you use a little oil, choose olive oil instead of the less flavorful vegetable oils.

- Heat oil thoroughly before sautéing food because cold oil is absorbed by the food more readily than hot oil.
- Avoid adding oil to marinades.
- Wrap fish in lettuce before baking to retain moisture. (Remove lettuce before serving—unless, of course, you love the taste of soggy, fishy lettuce!)
- To prevent yogurt from separating when heated, add one teaspoon of cornstarch for every cup of yogurt.
- Use yogurt, evaporated skim milk, or cottage cheese instead of cream.
- Vegetable purees can thicken sauces. Mashed or pureed potatoes make a good thickener.
- To sweeten dishes without table sugar or honey, use concentrated fruit juices such as frozen orange or apple juice.
- Substitute two egg whites for one whole egg.
- Add vegetables or pastas to meat dishes to decrease the amount of meat (and hence fat) per serving.

Certainly low-fat eating is very possible and possibly very tasty. On the other hand, berries do not quite match the taste sensations of cheesecakes or chocolate mousses. Grilled swordfish may be a real treat, but it does not rival the taste of a porterhouse steak. Unfortunately, high-fat food choices must become "alien food" to you if you expect to lose weight and keep it off forever. You *can* do it. Many, many thousands of people have made the switch to low-fat eating. It becomes a way of life, and it can be very satisfying. In any case, it beats the alternative for those of us who have lost weight. You cannot get to a lower weight and stay there without adopting a very low-fat eating plan.

The following *fat facts*, some of which have been reviewed in this chapter, underscore my emphasis on mastering this aspect of eating in order to lose weight and keep it off. Please review them carefully.

If you know your enemy (fat in this case) well, you can defeat it more readily.

- Your body uses very little energy to digest and store high-fat foods (for example, 3 calories of energy expended to digest 100 calories of bacon); your body uses much more energy to digest carbohydrates (22 calories expended to digest 100 calories of pasta).
- When you eat high-fat foods, the fat goes into storage very quickly—into your billions of hungry extra fat cells. When a never-overweight person eats high-fat foods, the fat goes into the muscles to be used as fuel.
- High-fat foods can cause an increase in appetite for more high-fat foods.
- Highly successful weight controllers report that their current successes, unlike prior weight losses, became permanent when they learned to eat very little fat.
- *Goal* for fat intake per day: as low as you can go (20 fat grams or less per day).

The following account provides an excellent example of how one of my clients focused his weight loss efforts on *very* low-fat eating. This focus led to great consistency and very satisfying long-term results.

John's Permanent 20-Pound Weight Loss: "It's My Body; That's the Way It Works."

John was forty-nine when we first met three years ago. He owned a successful, but very stressful, small business with forty employees and was happily married to his second wife, who was in a similar line of work. He lived primarily in Chicago but spent a lot of time commuting to a distant suburb, where his ex-wife and their two daughters lived. He also did considerable traveling for work. In fact, he estimated that he ate approximately one-third of his meals at restaurants.

John was quite happy in his work and with his second marriage (seven years at the time of our initial meeting). However, he was very dissatisfied with his weight and fitness levels. He had been used to living his life as a trim, five-foot-ten, 165-pound man who was fairly athletic. Over the past ten years, however, as his life had become more complex with more commuting and less available time, his exercising had become more sporadic and his weight had increased by 22 pounds. Although he was not substantially overweight, and the health risks of this amount of excess weight were modest, it really bothered him a great deal to feel as though he was in a body that, as he said, "wasn't right for me."

John's main barriers to successful and permanent weight control were:

- Inconsistent exercise (sometimes only once a week)
- Excessive drinking (one to two glasses of wine, sometimes much more, quite often)
- Often minimal eating early in the day or at midday, with excessive eating in the evening
- Some variability in consumption of fat (e.g., regular salad dressings on salads; bar food fairly often)

John had one perfect tendency for a weight controller: He liked looking at the details of his life. He was not at all adverse to monitoring, measuring, and focusing on exactly what he ate, how he exercised, and the circumstances that affected him either positively or negatively. He and I used this tendency to his advantage by encouraging him to use his computer to self-monitor (keep careful track of) his eating and exercising. He did this religiously and enjoyed the process. He also began incorporating a more consistent eating pattern, beginning in the morning and including a modest lunch. He loved and sought out vegetable sandwiches, essentially salads between two slices of bread, usually with mustard as a condiment.

John and I did not focus directly on decreasing his drinking, even though it might be a problem. He didn't want to modify his drinking and believed he could incorporate it at a moderate level into a healthy lifestyle.

The food records below were obtained approximately six months after John started his program with me. He had already lost all 22 pounds by this time, so these records suggest what worked for John (and what still works for him, three years after he began this effort). You will note in these records that he ate very limited amounts of fat. He and I both saw that as a critical aspect of his success. What does not appear in these records but was included in John's actual daily records was his exercising. This included at least 30 minutes of exercise virtually every single day—generally walking, running, using a treadmill, some weight lifting, and various stretching and related exercises.

Take a look at the following food records and consider what elements of John's approach you might incorporate into your own patterns. For example, you may wish to avoid using your calories for alcohol the way John does, but you might follow his example in minimizing your consumption of fat whenever and wherever possible.

Monday, October 6 / Weight: 165.0

		Calories	*Fat Grams*
7:00 A.M.	Coffee	25	0.5
	Banana-and-orange juice shake	165	1.0
12:00 Noon	Fruit	200	1.0
7:00 P.M.	Rice	200	0.0

	Calories	Fat Grams
Shrimp	90	1.0
Salmon	120	5.0
Pretzels	100	0.0
Wine	270	0.0
Milk	90	0.0
Frozen yogurt	120	0.0
Total	**1,380**	**8.5**

Tuesday, October 7 / Weight: 164.0

		Calories	Fat Grams
7:00 A.M.	Coffee	25	0.5
	Cereal	140	0.0
12:00 Noon	Veggie sandwich	180	1.5
	Turkey, 1 slice	20	0.5
8:00 P.M.	Veggies	100	2.0
	Mashed sweet potatoes	200	1.0
	Rolls	60	0.5
	Pretzels	100	0.0
	Frozen yogurt	120	0.0
	Milk	90	0.0
	Total	**1,035**	**6.0**

Saturday, October 11 / Weight: 164.5

		Calories	Fat Grams
7:00 A.M.	Cereal	140	0.0
	Coffee	25	0.5
12:00 Noon	Veggie sandwich	180	1.5
8:00 P.M.	Salad with clear rice noodles	100	0.0

	Calories	Fat Grams
Wine	180	0.0
Pretzels	100	0.0
Frozen Yogurt	120	0.0
Total	**845**	**2.0**

Sugar: How Sweet It Is—and Isn't

Happiness is the reward of an active life lived with "sweet reason," according to Aristotle. Writer Susan Cohler makes it clear why Americans often indulge in the sweet part of sweet reason:

> In the harsh light of the suburban ice cream parlor, a gangly adolescent creates a masterpiece. Three scoops of sweet delight nestled side by side, enfolded in the arms of a ripe banana. Steaming fudge drapes the ice cream slopes and snakes its way to the depths of the dish. A cloud of whipped cream, bejeweled with nuts and one cherry crowns the top. This ice cream treat is a work of edible art, but what it does to [you] . . . may be worth thinking about.

Sugar clearly permeates our lives. It can provide the foundation to "edible art," and it plays a major part in almost all of our celebrations (especially Valentine's Day, Easter, and Christmas). Think about the well-known phrases "Home sweet home" and "How sweet it is!" Think of many of the most common terms of endearment: sugar, sweetheart, sweetie, cookie, honeybunch, sugar plum, and sweet pea. I have personally used many of these terms to refer to my three young children. It makes me smile just to think of them with these phrases in mind, even as I write this sentence. Not only do our relationships involve sugar metaphors, but so do our sport performances. Have you seen a sports telecast that did *not* include such phrases as "sweet shot"? Sugar is idealized in these phrases. The best thing you can say about a person is that he or she is sweet.

Loving Sugar

What causes this infatuation with sugar? In fact, some biological roots may help explain it. When we are hungry, sugar provides the quickest antidote. In other words, the sugar you eat is very similar chemically to the primary source of energy in your body—glucose. Sugar is white, refined sucrose that is derived from sugarcane and beets. It is actually composed of glucose, in addition to fructose (fruit sugar). These components are readily split apart in the small intestine by the enzyme sucrase.

To take this example to its extreme, when humans or other animals are starving, they consistently show heightened preferences for very sweet foods. This, again, shows the body's orientation to satisfying extreme hunger and food deprivation quickly and effectively with sugar.

A second important factor reveals how sugar's appeal has biological roots: Sweet foods are safe foods. This harkens back to our earlier discussion of hunter-gatherers. Can you think of any examples of wild fruits or berries or vegetables that are sweet and also dangerous to eat? Probably not. If you find something hanging from a tree and it tastes sweet, it is almost certainly safe to eat. On the other hand, sour or bitter fruits or vegetables are much more likely to be poisonous.

A third factor that reveals the biological roots of sugar's appeal is the body's way of increasing the craving for sugar. The figure below illustrates one way it does this: When we eat carbohydrates, especially sugar, our production of insulin increases. Insulin directs glucose into our muscles and other organs. When we eat a sugary snack—a candy bar, for example—the body reacts to it by producing an excessive amount of insulin. This probably occurs because the body is programmed to eat large amounts of sugar or sweet foods whenever they are available. This made sense for hunter-gatherers; if they found something that tasted sweet, their bodies wanted to encourage them to eat large quantities of it. So when you eat that candy bar, your body is overprepared to digest it. This overpreparedness includes the release of an excess amount of insulin that clears the blood of most of its energy supply (glucose). There is now a very low level of glucose in the blood. The brain then detects this low level of glucose and causes a substantial increase in hunger. In other words, *when you eat sugary foods, it creates a biochemical chain reaction leading to increased hunger.*

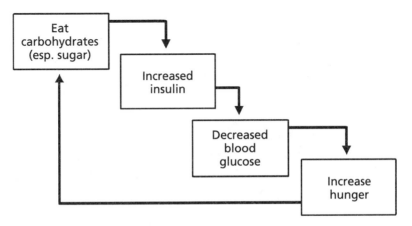

Fig. 3.2
Sugar Cycle and Weight Gain

The research that supports these assertions includes studies in which rabbits were fed glucose directly into their stomachs. These rabbits ate more, after receiving a high dose of sugar, than they did under normal conditions, and quite a bit more than rabbits who received only salt water injected into their stomachs. I've already discussed how fat begets fat; now you can see how sugar begets more sugar.

Mark, a very dedicated weight controller, tried to eat all the right things. Early on in his participation in my program, I noticed that he ate muesli regularly for breakfast. Muesli, granola, and similar cereals have a reputation for being health foods. After all, they are made from whole grains, contain lots of fiber, and are sold in health-food stores. Unfortunately, they contain lots of sugar. Sometimes the sugar is in the form of honey. But your body can't tell the difference between honey and sugar. Honey does contain small amounts of such minerals as potassium and calcium, but you would have to eat two hundred tablespoons of honey to meet the body's daily requirement for calcium.

I persuaded Mark that his muesli wasn't great for him. He substituted shredded wheat and was amazed that this simple change resulted in much less hunger throughout the day and dramatically decreased his cravings for sweets.

Recently, a new member joined the group in which Mark participated. Linda was eating low-fat granola for breakfast regularly. She also was snacking on candy bars later in the morning and sometimes in the afternoon as well. This pattern had contributed to significant weight gain over the past couple of years. Mark and I persuaded Linda to substitute a low-sugar food for her granola. Agreeing that "it's worth a shot," she began eating a bagel and low-fat cream cheese as an alternative to her usual breakfast of granola. She came back from this experiment saying, "The 'Muesli Syndrome' lives! I can't believe what a difference this made. I'm also amazed that it worked immediately. As soon as I started eating bagels instead of granola, I didn't have that gnawing feeling in my stomach at ten o'clock anymore. Wow!"

Energy Boost: Candy versus 10-Minute Walks

Robert Thayer, a California State University psychologist, conducted an important study demonstrating that sugar can also affect your mood. Thayer compared the effects of eating a ½ ounce candy bar (of any type) with those of taking a rapid 10-minute walk. When subjects took a 10-minute walk, their tension-level ratings decreased very quickly and, for two hours, stayed much lower than they were before the walk. In contrast, after they ate the candy bar, tension levels increased over a sixty-minute period and stayed high for the subsequent hour as well.

Similar effects occurred for ratings of energy levels. Subjects indicated feeling more energized for thirty minutes after eating the candy bar, but their energy levels fell to much lower levels one to two hours later. In contrast, when subjects took walks, their energy levels increased dramatically during the first thirty minutes and stayed well above their prewalk states for two hours afterward. Eating candy can cause a logy or tired feeling because it stimulates the release of a natural tranquilizer in our brains called serotonin.

These findings are very important. They suggest a good alternative to eating sugary snacks in order to feel energized. *A 10-minute brisk walk can provide a much better energy boost than a candy bar.* You won't find commercials encouraging people to take 10-minute walks for that "quick energy boost," though you will find plenty of commercials hawking candy bars for that purpose. Now you know the truth about which works better.

Conclusion

The moral of this story is: Avoid sugary foods. It is most helpful to avoid eating any foods as stand-alone snacks that contain lots of sugar, such as candy bars, ice cream cones, granola bars, caramel corn, and cookies. Some of these foods have tremendous nostalgic appeal. As Gail's story reveals, changing nostalgia-based food preferences can be very difficult.

It is also very wise to avoid sugary breakfast cereals. Instead, try low-sugar cereals, bagels, fruit, crackers, or raw vegetables. Also, try to take a brief walk to feel energized—sugar just makes you tired and hungry. This approach keeps the blood glucose levels relatively stable. It also helps avoid some of the other chemical reactions that produce strong cravings for some very high-calorie (and high-fat) foods.

Gail's Christmas-Cookie Tradition

Gail began working with me on a major effort to lose weight six years ago and continues attending weekly group meetings as of this writing. Gail is a forty-two-year-old high school teacher and a dedicated mother of two children. She had gained fifty pounds gradually over twelve years and two pregnancies, during a hectic (but sedentary) life.

Gail became intensively energized during a classic Honeymoon stage when she first came to our group. She monitored her eating and exercising meticulously and focused beautifully. She varied her exercising, starting with slow but consistent walking and experimenting with racquetball and swimming. She modified her eating to include primarily foods that were low in fat and sugar. Gail lapsed occasionally by eating cookies and other sweets, but she took these lapses in stride and kept moving forward persistently.

Then, six months into her Honeymoon, after losing twenty-eight pounds, came Christmas. "I've got to make my cookies!" she reported.

"What do you mean 'got to'? And how many cookies are you talking about, anyway?" I asked.

"I mean I've *got to* make these cookies. It's a wonderful tradition in my family. It's one of the few traditions that my mother established when I was growing up. We all looked forward to it. It's a neat project for families. The kids create their own decorations. It's creative and important. We make many batches, dozens and dozens of cookies. Then we mail them out and give them out as presents."

Gail certainly was committed to those cookies—to lots and lots of those cookies! Unfortunately, cookies are committed to fat cells and increasing hunger (for more cookies, especially if two hundred or so are sitting around "smiling" enticingly).

Gail, her group, and I talked about this dilemma. There was no simple solution. I emphasized the biology of weight control.

The group talked about using alternative artsy projects for kids. They encouraged Gail to start a new, lower-calorie tradition; they talked about spreading "the word" to friends and relatives about sugar. But how can your words encourage people to reduce consumption of sugar (and fat), when your deeds (giving the cookies) say the opposite?

Gail reacted emotionally to the idea of giving up her cookie tradition. She *couldn't* get herself to do it, she claimed. But she did decrease the amount of cookies she and her children baked and gave away. She also wound up munching on "too many cookies."

The next year Gail vacillated between the Frustration and Acceptance stages. She baked very few cookies during her third year in the program (but still munched on too many). Finally, the cookie tradition was replaced with the computer-generated "artistic greeting-card tradition."

Gail has now lost most of the fifty pounds that she had gained over the years. She still vacillates between Frustration and Acceptance, but she spends far more time in Acceptance these days. She still munches on "too many cookies" sometimes, but avoids placing herself directly in harm's way by refusing to bake dozens of cookies for Christmas. Her weight fluctuates more than she would like. She persists.

Specific Eating Plans

How do you take the ideas of striving for 20 fat grams or less and limiting sugar to build an eating plan that works for you? Let's consider some principles and plans that can help you do just that. First, take a look at the very first diet that became remarkably popular in the middle to latter part of the nineteenth century, Banting's 1863 Diet.

Banting's 1863 Diet:
The World's First Bestselling Diet
How Times Have Changed—
and How Times Have Not Changed

The following excerpt is from the first popular booklet on dieting, *Letter on Corpulence, Addressed to the Public,* by William Banting (published in Kensington, England, in December 1863).

Of all the parasites that affect humanity I do not know of, nor can I imagine, any more distressing than that of obesity, and, having just emerged from a very long probation in this affliction, I am desirous of circulating my humble knowledge and experience for the benefit of my fellow man, with an earnest hope it may lead to the same comfort and happiness I now feel under the extraordinary change—which might almost be termed miraculous had it not been accomplished by the most simple common-sense means.

For the sake of argument and illustration I will presume that certain articles of ordinary diet, however beneficial in youth, are prejudicial in advanced life, like beans to a horse, whose common ordinary food is hay and corn. It may be useful food occasionally, under peculiar circumstances, but detrimental as a constancy. I will, therefore, adopt the analogy, and call such food human beans. The items from which I was advised (by my physician, Dr. William Harvey) to abstain as much as possible were: bread, butter, milk, sugar, beer, and potatoes, which had been the main (and I thought innocent) elements of my existence, or at all events they had for many years been adopted freely.

These, said my excellent adviser, contain starch and saccharine matter, tending to create fat, and should be avoided altogether. At the first blush it seemed to me that I had little left to live upon, but my kind friend soon showed me there was ample, and I was only too happy to give the plan a fair trial, and, within a very few days, found immense benefit from it. It may better elucidate the dietary plan if I describe generally what I have sanction to take, and that man must be an extraordinary person who would desire a better table.

For breakfast, I take four or five ounces of beef, mutton, kidneys, broiled fish, bacon, or cold meat of any kind except pork; a large cup of tea (without milk or sugar), a little biscuit, or one ounce of dry toast.

For dinner, five or six ounces of any fish except salmon, any meat except pork, any vegetable except potato, one ounce of dry toast, fruit out of a pudding, any kind of poultry or game, and two or three glasses of good claret, sherry, or Madeira—Champagne, Port and beer forbidden.

For tea, two or three ounces of fruit, a rusk or two, and a cup of tea without milk or sugar.

For supper, three or four ounces of meat or fish, similar to dinner, with a glass or two of claret.

For nightcap, if required, a tumbler of grog—(gin, whisky, or brandy, without sugar)—or a glass or two of claret or sherry.

This plan leads to an excellent night's rest, with from six to eight hours' sound sleep. The dry toast or rusk may have a tablespoonful of spirit to soften it, which will prove acceptable. Perhaps I did not wholly escape starchy or saccharine matter, but scrupulously avoided those beans, such as milk, sugar, beer, butter, & c., which were known to contain them.

Experience has taught me to believe that these human beans are the most insidious enemies man, with a tendency to corpulence in advanced life, can possess, though eminently friendly to youth. He may very prudently mount guard against such an enemy if he is not a fool to himself, and I fervently hope this truthful unvarnished tale may lead him to make a trial of my plan, which I sincerely recommend to public notice,—not with any ambitious motive, but in sincere good faith to help my fellow-creatures to obtain the marvelous blessings I have found within the short period of a few months.

I have not felt so well as now for the last twenty years.

Have suffered no inconvenience whatever in the probational remedy.

Am reduced many inches in bulk, and 35 lbs. in weight in thirty-eight weeks.

Come down stairs forward naturally, with perfect ease.

Go up stairs and take ordinary exercise freely, without the slightest inconvenience.

Can perform every necessary office for myself.

The umbilical rupture is greatly ameliorated, and gives me no anxiety.

My sight is restored—my hearing improved.

My other bodily ailments are ameliorated; indeed, almost past into matter of history.

William Banting sought only to relieve "suffering humanity" by distributing the dietary plan to which he attributed his successful weight reduction. His booklet on the subject was reprinted ten times, and more than one hundred thousand copies of it were distributed free or sold. It met with great enthusiasm and tremendous controversy as well. Many people expressed outrage about even discussing obesity and weight control. For example, an editorial appearing in the January 25, 1865, issue of *Commercial Advertiser* exclaimed:

> Good heavens! The ill of the world is not repletion. It is emptiness and all the other fat men are running about in their own puffery and breathless manner asking: What about malt? How is it as to chocolate? Are anchovies bad for me? Must I cut off my Stilton? To these I say: Let me be your doctor. Retrench your all-absorbing self interest. Turn your thoughts from your duodenum to the famishing creatures who peer down through the railings of your areas at the blazing fire in your kitchen grate. Give up this filthy selfishness that takes for its worship all that is least worthy in humanity. Walk, ride, bathe, swim, fast if you must, but take your thoughts off this detestable theme and try to remember that the subject you want to popularize is in its details one of the coarsest that can be made matter for conversation.

William Banting's motives were pure, but his Banting System created a great moral controversy. The dietary plan he recommended was based on some notions from the mid–nineteenth century about the manner in which the liver works. The actual dietary plan emphasized protein intake in accord with these views. The Banting System recommends consuming more than twice as much protein as the current dietary recommendations endorsed by the U.S. Department of Agriculture. Many subsequent bestsellers also emphasize high-protein diets. Very few current dietary plans suggest consuming

23 percent of one's calories in alcohol! The Banting System did this. Quite a remarkable recommendation, by today's standards of health.

The "Almost Never" Plan

"I know what to do, it's getting myself to do it—that's the problem."

I've heard this statement and versions of it hundreds of times. Scientific research also supports it. Studies show that when weight controllers begin a program, regardless of its content, they often make healthful changes in their eating and exercising habits. Yet most people don't understand *the degree to which certain of the rules apply*. For example, how many people really have a complete understanding of some of the biological forces that make weight control so challenging? Most people do not appreciate the degree to which fat and sugar present major biological challenges. Also, highly successful weight controllers say that their current success occurred only because they became more strict in limiting their eating to very low-fat foods. Because of this, I find it is helpful to state very clearly some rules to live by for effective weight control: the "Almost Never" rules—types of food to avoid as much as possible, and the "Almost Always" rules—principles of eating to follow as much as possible.

Effective weight control happens when weight controllers eat the following foods and preparations "almost never." Occasional, very rare consumption of these foods and types of food preparations is expected. But *each incident* in which these foods are eaten is best viewed as a problem. It is not sinful, shameful, horrible, or awful to deviate from this plan; the deviations are simply problems to be solved. Successful weight controllers solve these problems well and strive very consistently to "almost never" consume the foods on this list.

Almost Never Eat:
- Fried foods (except no-oil stir-fries)
- Desserts, other than fruit or very low-fat alternatives

- High-fat lunch meats (bologna, salami)
- Candy (candy bars, truffles)—regular-fat kinds
- Regular salad dressings
- High-fat cookies, brownies, cake
- Mayonnaise (except fat-free mayonnaise)
- Cheese (other than no-fat or very low-fat cheese, 2 grams of fat per ounce or less)
- High-fat ice cream and ice cream products (milkshakes, malts)
- High-fat gravy and other high-fat sauces

Almost Always Eat:
- Low-fat, low-sugar foods
- Low-fat, low-sugar snacks (popcorn, pretzels, fruit, rice cakes, low-calorie and low-fat cocoa, Jell-O, puddings)
- Grilled fish and fowl
- Vegetables
- Salads (dressing on the side, preferably low-calorie and low-fat)
- Mustard or ketchup or barbecue sauce on sandwiches
- Spicy foods
- Salsa on practically everything
- Pastas (with tomato sauces or plain)

Weight controllers often ask questions like the following ones after reviewing these "Almost Always" and "Almost Never" principles.

Question: What about pizza? Pizza, after all, has all of the food groups.

Answer: Pizzas often contain vegetables, dairy, meat, and grains, and they do, indeed, provide a wide range of food groups. This fact would be very important if you were starving on a desert island. However, pizza also contains many calories, and many of those calories come from fat. For example, a two-slice serving of a national fast food pizza chain's stuffed pizza contains 860 calories and 40 grams of fat (42 percent of the calories come from fat). Even this pizza chain's less caloric pizzas, as well as the largest national chain's full range of pizza offerings, contain 30 to 50 percent of their calories from fat. Pizza cheese (mozzarella), made with part-skim milk, is *still* a high-fat food, and pizzas generally have a lot of cheese on them.

The good news is that many places will serve pizzas without any cheese, which does represent a reasonable food choice. The crust in some pizzas contains some fat (usually 1 to 2 grams per slice), but as an alternative food, pizzas with no cheese can work quite well.

If you are trapped in a meeting and surrounded by pizzas, what can you do? You can perform minor surgery and remove the cheese from your pizza. Some people may find this distasteful, and although it is not the most acceptable form of behavior, it could work a lot better for you than eating high-fat food and interfering with your efforts at effective weight control.

Question: What about frozen yogurt?

Answer: Many frozen yogurts fit into the low-fat "Almost Always" category. However, some of them can be surprisingly high in fat content and, therefore, come close to violating the "Almost Never" rule for ice cream. If you are selective and read labels carefully, you can find low-fat or no-fat frozen yogurts. But remember that most frozen yogurts contain lots of sweeteners, and this could trigger some of the same reactions that other sugary foods do.

Many weight controllers use frozen yogurt in modest amounts as a treat, which is a good approach. Just be careful of establishments that serve nearly twice the amounts that they advertise for a given price. Try ordering the smallest, child-size portion available at a frozen yogurt stand or restaurant. Frozen yogurt can also become problematic if it is purchased in pints, quarts, or larger bulk quantities. Many people find themselves dipping into these treats more often than desirable. So the answer is: Use frozen yogurt with caution.

Question: What about birthday cake?

Answer: Birthday cakes are an important tradition to many people. However, traditions can change. Why would you want to eat a food that creates a problem for you in celebration of a special day? When you first had a birthday cake to celebrate your birthday during childhood, you didn't realize the kind of problem that foods high in sugar and fat create for you. In fact, at that time, you probably didn't have such a problem. Now you have new information that advises against consuming foods like cake. In the 1950s, practically every dinner table in America had red meat on it, but that tradition has changed. In William Banting's day (mid-1800s), drinking liberal quantities of alcohol was traditional. That tradition has also changed. It is now time for you to consider changing the birthday cake tradition for yourself. This position may seem rather extreme, but weight control takes extreme focusing and persistence. If you really want to succeed at this difficult challenge, you must take difficult steps.

Another problem with allowing yourself birthday cake is that if you give yourself permission for this deviation from the plan, what else will you permit? What about other holidays? What about other people's birthdays? What about your children's birthdays? Some of the clients with whom I have worked give themselves permission to eat problematic foods when they are hungry, tired, on vacation, at someone else's house for dinner or for a party, or when they are sad or depressed. The list goes on and on.

Permissions often create problems. For example, if you give yourself permission to eat problematic food today, then you may struggle mightily with other food decisions tomorrow. These struggles take their toll. Instead of food becoming more secondary in your life, the struggle becomes primary. Lots of struggles can put you into a major Frustration stage—an unpleasant stage that often produces unfavorable results. Can all of these problems come from a birthday cake? Perhaps!

Question: How can you tell about sauces in restaurants?

Answer: You can assume that any sauce made in a restaurant with oil as a primary ingredient is problematic. On the other hand, tomato sauces and sauces that are essentially broths (which are available increasingly in restaurants) are quite acceptable. Any sauces made with cheese (such as Alfredo sauce) are very high in fat; similarly, sauces and soups with cream bases are very high-fat foods.

One of my clients recently told a story about a seemingly innocuous mushroom soup that her dining companion ordered. Her companion raved about how wonderful the soup was, and it looked very appealing to the client. But when she tasted the soup, she soon realized that its primary ingredient was butter. The word "mushroom" suggests a low-fat, safe, vegetable base. As Americans become increasingly health-conscious, restaurateurs and food packagers will market and name products to suggest their healthfulness. You can generally assume that if you're not sure about the ingredients in a product, it's best to avoid it. In a restaurant, try to order only items for which you know the fat and sugar contents. These guidelines may sound stringent, but unfortunately, your biology demands such stringencies. Successful weight controllers follow these guidelines with tremendous consistency.

Most diets provide numerous recipes. Because recipes are often detailed and sometimes hard to follow, people do not use them very much. The central ideas in the recipes can, however, provide helpful guidance about low-fat and low-sugar meals. Breakfast and lunch are less challenging for most weight controllers than dinner. No-fat cereals that have no sugar or very little sugar, mixed with skim milk, and bagels or low-calorie bread and no-fat cheese are simple and effective breakfasts. Common lunches include turkey or chicken sandwiches, salads with low-fat dressing, broth-based soups, and fruit. In the United States, dinners and the evening generally present the biggest challenge for weight controllers. People relax more in the evening, decrease their focus on goals, and eat in a more elaborate and leisurely manner than they do during the day.

My clients use the ideas presented in the following list to help them follow the principles of the "Almost Never" plan during the challenging times of the day. You will notice that the list focuses on central ideas about meals rather then presenting highly specific formulas for how to prepare them. You might find this approach more useful than the usual method of presenting recipes. If you take the ideas and experiment with them to make them your own, you will build your own set of mainstay meals for dinner based on the "Almost Never" plan. These meals, and this approach more generally, will produce not only improved weight control, but improved health.

Eating and Cancer:
Can You Prevent Cancer by Eating Better?

Cancer strikes 10 million people a year. But 3 to 4 million of those cancers could have been prevented through healthier eating and exercising. In fact, eating more fruits and vegetables alone could eliminate as many as 2 million new cases of cancer a year.

In 1997, the World Cancer Research Fund and the American Institute for Cancer Research issued a comprehensive report on the relationship between eating and cancer. This report, based on a careful review of more than 4,500 studies, stressed that no food or drink can prevent cancer but concluded that a diet that emphasizes certain foods can certainly lower your risk of getting this deadly disease.

Five eating and drinking strategies that almost certainly can decrease the risk of getting cancer are:

1. *Eat lots of* VEGETABLES. The average American eats only three or four servings a day of vegetables and fruits. Five servings are clearly preferable, and nine are recommended by virtually all nutritional experts. Yellow, dark green, and orange vegetables rich in carotenoids and the cabbage family vegetables (broccoli, brussels sprouts, cauliflower, collards, kale, bok choy, and mustard and turnip greens) all seem to lower the risk of cancer. Garlic, onions, and leeks may also help ward off cancer, especially breast cancer.

2. *Eat Lots of* FRUITS. Fruits that are rich in vitamin C (all citrus fruits, tomatoes, and strawberries) are especially helpful.

3. *Decrease consumption of total* FAT, *particularly saturated fat.* The panel recommended that fats should provide between 15 and 30 percent of total calories. You may recall that I have recommended that you go "as low as you can go" in total fat. For most, this may amount to 10 percent (or slightly more) of your total calories in fat.

4. *Decrease* ALCOHOL *consumption; limit drinks to less than two a day for men and one a day for women.* The panel concluded that although alcohol may have some benefits for decreasing heart disease when consumed in small amounts, the risk for cancers, particularly breast, colon, and rectal cancers, is significant. People who consume even small amounts of alcohol show a significantly greater chance of developing cancer than those who do not drink alcohol at all.

5. *The following other foods and drinks may also help reduce the risk of cancer, at least somewhat: dried beans, milk, fish, green*

tea, whole-grain cereals, and olive oil. The evidence favoring these particular foods and drinks is not as convincing as the evidence in the first four recommendations. Nonetheless, the panel concluded that these items may prove beneficial and are worth including in healthy eating plans.

Favorite Dinner Ideas from the "Almost Never" Plan

Frozen grain-based ground-beef imitators. This type of pseudo-beef is available in frozen food sections. It usually contains 0 to 3 grams of fat per serving and far fewer calories than ground beef. Use it to make tacos and chili.

- Tacos: Combine (for one serving) 4 ounces of very lean ground beef, imitation ground beef, or 99 percent fat-free ground turkey with a taco seasoning packet in a nonstick frying pan (no need to add oil). Add canned tomatoes if desired. After cooking, add fresh chopped vegetables (for example, bell peppers, lettuce, cucumbers, tomatoes) and salsa. Serve over Spanish rice or in flour or corn tortilla shells.
- Chili: Combine with light red kidney beans, canned tomatoes, chili, onion powder, and garlic. For four servings, use 16 ounces of very lean ground beef, turkey, or soybean meat substitute, and freeze leftovers. Serve over macaroni.

Pasta. Combine any type of pasta with fat-free tomato sauce. Combine them with one whole or one-half can of clams and use salsa if desired.

Baked white and sweet potatoes. Bake in a microwave and combine with no-fat or 1 percent cottage cheese or plain yogurt and broccoli and salsa, if desired. Or consider melting no-fat mozzarella cheese on top.

Grilled vegetables. Very lightly coat any vegetables (for example, carrots, peppers, zucchini, onions, potatoes) with olive oil or, better yet, flavored vinegar and broil with garlic. Cook a large quantity and eat with no-fat or low-fat yogurt.

Stir-fries. Use cilantro, garlic, and parsley, and experiment with a variety of other spices to create seasonings (for example, consider using dried red peppers and sliced ginger to create particularly spicy dishes). Stir-fry in water or fat-free broths, or use Pam or other no-fat cooking agents. Combine with frozen, peeled shrimp and an assortment of vegetables. Serve over rice. Turkey breast or chicken breast without skin can be substituted for the shrimp. It helps to get a wok with a Teflon or other nonstick cooking surface.

Frozen entrées and low-fat soups. Check ingredients carefully and combine these minimeals with fresh salads and fruit. Healthy Choice soups and a wide variety of frozen dinners work well. Soups from Asian restaurants can often fit this plan (e.g., in Thai restaurants try tom-yum soup; for Chinese dinners, choose yat gaw mein or hot and sour).

The Popcorn Plan

The Popcorn Plan encourages people to use popcorn (preferably air-popped) as an evening snack. Popcorn provides a tasty treat and dietary fiber (3.1 grams for 3 cups) at a cost of relatively few calories and a small amount of fat. For example, 3 cups of air-popped popcorn contain 75 calories and approximately 2 grams of fat. A typical bag of "light" (low-fat) microwaved popcorn has 200 calories and 7 fat grams (6 cups popped).

Three cups of popcorn is one of the selections in the following list of breads and starches. This plan includes seven selections of proteins, five selections of breads and starches, two fruits, and unlimited vegetables. There are also some foods, listed under a miscellaneous heading, that you can consume as desired, with a few exceptions. The following table summarizes the plan.

Group	Servings per Day
Proteins	7
Breads and starches	5
Fruits	2
Free vegetables	As much as desired
Miscellaneous	As much as desired (with some exceptions as noted)

Food selections are listed on the following pages. You will see that quite a wide variety of foods are available on this plan. However, all foods are to be prepared without any butter or oils. Food preparation is limited to steaming, broiling, grilling, no-fat stir-frying, and other methods that add no extra calories.

The Popcorn Plan provides approximately 1,000 calories per day. It encourages a style of eating that provides very modest amounts of fat (less than 20 fat grams per day). Three sample menus follow the lists of food groups and supplements.

Proteins (7 servings per day)

1 serving = 1 ounce; approximately 50 calories; 0–2 fat grams

Chicken breast without skin and trimmed of fat	1 oz.
Cheese (no-fat)	1 oz.
Cottage cheese (1% fat)	¼ cup
Egg whites	2; cook with Pam
Fish (including shellfish), any kind (e.g., tuna, swordfish, clams, shrimp, lobster, catfish, scallops, cod, flounder)	1 oz.
Skim milk	¾ cup
Turkey breast without skin	1 oz.
Veal, dark meat of chicken	Limit to 2 servings per week

Breads and Starches (5 servings per day)

1 serving = 1 selection; approximately 80 calories; less than 1 fat gram

Breads

Bagel	½ small
Bialy	1
White (also French and Italian)	1 slice
Whole wheat	1 slice
Rye or pumpernickel	1 slice
Raisin (no icing)	1 slice
Bread crumbs, dry	3 Tbs.
Bread sticks (7 in. long × ¾ in. diameter)	4
Bun, hamburger or hot dog	½
Croutons, plain	½ cup
English muffin	½ small
Melba toast, oblong	4
Melba toast, round	8
Pita (8 in. diameter)	½
Rolls, pan or hard	½ large, 1 small
Rusk	2
Tortilla, corn or flour (6 in. diameter)	1

Cereals

Cooked	½ cup
Grits	½ cup
Ready-to-eat, dry and no sugar coating	¾ cup
Bran, all types but check calories	⅓ to ⅔ cup
Grape-Nuts	3 Tbs.
Puffed wheat or puffed rice	1 cup
Shredded wheat biscuits	1 large or ½ cup spoon-size

Starchy vegetables

Baked beans, no pork	¼ cup
Corn, whole kernel	⅓ cup
Corn, ear (4 in. long)	1
Popcorn (air-popped)	3 cups
Dried beans and peas, cooked	½ cup
Lentils	½ cup
Lima beans	½ cup
Mixed vegetables	½ cup
Parsnips	⅔ cup
Peas, green	½ cup
Potato, white	1 small, ½ cup mashed
Potato, sweet, or yam	¾ cup
Pumpkin	¾ cup
Squash: acorn, rhubarb, butternut	½ cup

Note: I recommend that you have popcorn for one of your selections every day.

Crackers

Matzo (6 in. square)	1
Oyster	20 or ½ cup
Rye wafers (2 in. × 3½ in.)	3
Saltines	6
Soda (2½ in. square)	4
Zwieback	2

Pastas and Grains

Barley, pearl, dry	1½ Tbs.
Macaroni, cooked	½ cup
Noodles, cooked	½ cup
Rice, cooked	½ cup
Spaghetti or other pasta, cooked	½ cup
Wheat germ	¼ cup

Fruits (2 servings per day)

1 serving = 80 calories; 1 fat gram or less

Any type. The most desirable (for potassium needs) are grapefruit, banana, cantaloupe, and nectarine.

Free vegetables

Raw or steamed and eat as much as you'd like

Alfalfa sprouts	Broccoli
Cabbage	Cauliflower
Celery	Chicory
Chinese cabbage	Chives
Cucumbers	Endive
Escarole	Lettuce
Mushrooms	Parsley
Peppers	Radishes
Zucchini	Spinach
	Watercress

Miscellaneous

Use or eat as desired unless otherwise noted

Baking Aids

Baking powder	Baking soda
Cream of tartar	Flavoring extracts, pure
Yeast, baking	

Beverages

Clam juice (limit to ½ cup per day)	Club soda
Coffee	Decaffeinated coffee
Decaffeinated tea	Carbonated water
Mineral water	Postum (limit to 1 tsp. per meal)
Sugar-free carbonated drinks	Sauerkraut juice (limit to 1 cup per day)

Condiments

Artificial sweetener

Hot pepper sauce

Mustard, prepared

Pimento

Tabasco sauce

Vinegar

Herbed vinegar

Horseradish

Pickles, unsweetened

Salsa

Taco sauce

Worcestershire sauce

Soups

Beef tea

Broth, without fat

Bouillon cubes, prepared with
  water

Seasonings

Celery seeds or celery salt

Herbs (e.g., sage, oregano,
  thyme, basil)

Mustard, dry

Paprika

Poppy seeds

Salt, seasoned salt,
  salt substitutes

Tenderizers

Garlic, garlic powder, garlic salt,
  garlic juice

Mint leaves

Onion salt, onion powder, onion
  flakes, onion juice

Pepper

Poultry seasoning

Spices (e.g., cloves, cinnamon,
  ginger, cumin)

Limit to 2 tbs. per day

Chili sauce, without sugar

Cocoa, dry unsweetened
  powder

Salad dressings—only those
  with 20 calories or
  less per tbs. (no-fat
  preferred)

Yeast, brewer's

Cocktail sauce

Jam and jelly, artificially
  sweetened

Soy sauce

Other

Cranberries, unsweetened

Gelatin, unflavored or artificially
  sweetened

Lemon (limit to 1 per day or
  ¼ cup juice per day)

Lime (limit to 2 per day
  or ¼ cup juice per day)

Here are three sample menus that follow the Popcorn Plan. You can get as creative as possible to add variety. Greater variety often leads to greater satisfaction.

Sample Menu #1

. . . .

Breakfast
: ½ bagel (or 1 bialy)
  2 oz. lox

Snack
: Celery and cucumber slices

Lunch
: 2 oz. tuna with fat-free salad dressing
  ¾ cup skim milk
  Salad: lettuce, cucumber, green pepper,
    tomatoes with vinegar, lemon juice, or
    1 Tbs. of no-oil dressing
  ½ slice rye toast

Snack
: Radishes, zucchini slices, 1 apple

Dinner
: 3 oz. bass with lemon juice, parsley flakes,
    and garlic powder
  1 medium baked potato
  Salad: sliced fresh mushrooms on a bed of
    raw fresh spinach sprinkled with herbed
    vinegar or lemon juice
  ¾ cup skim milk
  1 orange

Snack
: 3 cups air-popped or light popcorn

Sample Menu #2

. . . .

Breakfast	3-egg-white omelet with ½ cup cottage cheese (1% fat), onion, and green pepper
	1 slice cracked-wheat bread
	1 grapefruit
Snack	Celery sticks
Lunch	1 cup broth or bouillon (chicken, beef, or vegetable)
	2 oz. shrimp and 1 oz. turkey breast on romaine lettuce with alfalfa sprouts, green pepper, tomato, celery, and 1 Tbs. of fat-free dressing
	1 slice cracked-wheat bread
Snack	Cucumber slices, 1 apple
Dinner	3 oz. broiled whitefish or swordfish with lemon, rosemary, sage, and thyme
	1 cup rice
	Salad: raw cabbage with 1 Tbs. of fat-free dressing, vinegar, or lemon juice and celery salt, onion salt or powder, and/or dill
Snack	3 cups of air-popped or light popcorn

Sample Menu #3

. . . .

Breakfast	½ English muffin with ¼ cup of cottage cheese (1%) and cinnamon, broiled
	1 banana
Snack	1 oz. turkey
	Lettuce leaves
Lunch	1 cup broth

	3 oz. veal sautéed (with Pam) with lemon juice, garlic, and basil
Snack	Green pepper slices, 1 apple
Dinner	3 oz. broiled scallops with lemon
	½ cup peas
	Salad: spinach, alfalfa sprouts, and raw zucchini with 1 Tbs. fat-free dressing
	1 slice Italian bread
	¾ cup skim milk
Snack	3 cups of air-popped or light popcorn

Every basic eating plan has a foundation. The Popcorn Plan, like all structured eating plans or diets, may help you stay within the boundaries of the "Almost Never" principles. Many of my clients have used this plan as a skeleton around which they have constructed their own style of eating. That approach makes sense. There is no value in beating yourself up for not following relatively arbitrary rules. For example, would it really matter if you had six proteins instead of seven and with six servings of starch instead of five? The answer is no. Perhaps the Popcorn Plan can help you develop your own approach. The key to making this work is to provide yourself with some leeway. It may help you to have a structure, but it will certainly hurt you if you become very critical and unforgiving about a reasonable amount of deviation from that structure.

Does Eating Right Cost Too Much?

Do you think that buying fresh fruits and vegetables, even in the dead of winter, will empty your bank account? Researchers have found that four out of ten people believe that buying fruits, vegetables, fish, and other healthful foods, particularly out of season, costs more than the items they currently buy. But this is just not true.

When researchers gave several hundred people with high cholesterol levels videos that showed them how to cut fat from their diets, those whose cholesterol levels dropped the most after nine months also decreased their food bills by more than a dollar a day (on average). If a family of four were to follow this pattern, that family would save $1,600 per year.

Consider the cost differences between a doughnut or a muffin bought at a convenience store and cereal with skim milk. The cereal and skim milk will cost quite a bit less than the surprisingly pricey bakery goods. Consider another example: Do you think twice about spending three dollars on a pint of your favorite pseudo-imported frozen yogurt? What about spending the same three dollars for a pint of strawberries in the dead of winter to top that frozen yogurt? You may resist spending money for the strawberries, but not for the frozen yogurt. Compare the three dollars spent on the frozen yogurt or on a grande latte versus three dollars for six frozen veggie burgers.

Even if your appetite tends toward rather pricey fruits and vegetables in the off-season, consider how much time, energy, and money you put into the effort to stay healthy and lose weight. Isn't that asparagus worth it? Aren't you worth it?

F O U R

❖

Focusing Clearly

Truth #6: If you maintain a written record of your eating and exercising at least 75 percent of the time, you can manage the program successfully.

Consider any diet that you've tried. Perhaps it involved eating more protein and counting grams of protein consumed. Perhaps it involved eating unlimited portions of a special soup. Perhaps it involved eating certain combinations of foods at certain times of day. Perhaps it involved attempting to eliminate fat and counting fat grams. Perhaps it involved following a plan using foods provided for you.

What did the diet do for you? Did it

- help you eliminate certain types of problematic foods?
- give you hope?
- help you focus on this issue in your life?
- help you reduce the total amount of food you ate?
- increase your awareness about eating and exercising?

Every diet shares these features. It really doesn't matter what the diet meant to accomplish or how. Most of the effects of traditional diets, at least most of the initial beneficial effects, happen because these specific food plans help you concentrate, reduce your total intake of food, and improve your motivation. If the "magic" was something specific about the diet—certain combinations of foods, for example—then how could so many bestsellers suggest radically different approaches?

Let's consider some interesting examples. You may recall from a previous chapter the very first diet ever published, William Banting's *Letter on Corpulence* (printed in England in 1863). Remember that although the term "Banting System" became synonymous with "diet" for several decades in the late 1800s, this method recommended consuming twice as much protein as suggested by modern nutritionists. It also advocated drinking 23 percent of one's calories from alcohol! The Banting System seems very quaint by today's standards, yet it was widely accepted for many decades as the best way to lose weight.

The account on the following page describes what has become the most popular dietary recommendation in many years, Barry Sears's *The Zone*. *The Zone*'s approach, which has spawned many follow-up books, makes about as much sense as the Banting System. Yet Americans have sworn by this latest diet craze.

The assertions in *The Zone* seem much more scientifically credible in the late twentieth century than Banting's mid–nineteenth-century ideas. Despite the fact that the book was written by a man with a Ph.D. (who has, however, never published a single article in a professional journal on weight loss), the scientific evidence supports Banting's approach just as "well" as it supports *The Zone*. For example, *The Zone*'s author, Barry Sears, argues that because we Americans now eat *less fat* than we used to, we have caused ourselves to become *fatter*. Contrary to Sears's claim, research shows that we Americans eat *more*, not less, fat than we used to (83 fat grams per day now versus 81 grams twenty years ago). How could eating *less* fat in recent years (something that didn't happen) explain America's weight gain?

A Modern Diet Craze: The Zone

Barry Sears's *The Zone* has sold millions of copies, as have its more recent sequels. The book makes several surprising assertions. It uses scientific language and stresses repeatedly that tremendous amounts of scientific data support each of the following propositions:

- Americans are gaining excess weight because we are eating *less* fat.
- By eating too many carbohydrates (like rice, potatoes, pasta), we send a hormonal message, via insulin, to the body saying, "Store fat."
- Calories and fat don't count; protein does.
- Virtually every disease (including heart disease, cancer, arthritis, and multiple sclerosis) can be viewed as caused by the body making more bad eicosanoids and too few good eicosanoids. (Eicosanoids are hormones that help regulate inflammation, blood clotting, and the immune system.)

Do you believe these assertions?

These assertions are probably false. For example, Americans now eat slightly more fat, not less, than we did twenty years ago. A much more reasonable explanation for the increase in weight by Americans has to do with continuing to eat too much fat while eating too many calories (100 to 300 more than twenty years ago) and getting too little exercise. Sears's other claims, such as the notion that eating carbohydrates causes obesity and that eating equal amounts of carbohydrates and protein somehow decreases obesity, also have no reasonable scientific basis.

Diets Don't Work

Consider the logic of the following recommendations from some recent bestsellers:

- Virtually eliminate potatoes, corn, white rice, bread from refined flour, beets, carrots, and, of course, refined sugar, corn syrup, molasses, honey, sugared colas, and beer.

- Never let yourself get hungry; stop worrying about fat; and plan your meals around the right number of grams of protein.
- Eat whatever "extras" you want (including very high-fat meats and desserts), but avoid bananas, cherries, grapes, dried fruits, and pineapple.
- Discontinue eating chicken and turkey sandwiches because eating proteins and carbohydrates together puts a strain on the digestive system.
- Eat "balanced reward meals" every day, including proteins, vegetables, and carbohydrates (including desserts) arranged on a plate by volume so that each type of food occupies one-third of the plate.
- Eat equal amounts of proteins and carbohydrates at every meal.
- Use an individualized diet based on whether your blood type is O, A, B, or AB.
- Forget about calories! Don't even think about calories.

From a scientific standpoint, none of these recommendations makes any sense. Yet this is the stuff that fills bestselling books claiming to have discovered the latest and best way to lose weight. Science tells us, science shouts at us, to ignore the advice contained in these diets.

Self-Monitoring Does Work

Self-monitoring is the careful observation and recording of behavior that you wish to change. For weight controllers, self-monitoring involves observing and recording eating and exercising behaviors.

Most experts on helping people lose weight agree on at least one thing: *Self-monitoring is the single most important aspect of effective weight control.* The list on pages 87 and 88 was created using scientific research that clearly makes this point. The studies reviewed for the list show that when people write down at least 75 percent of their eating and exercising behaviors they often succeed in losing weight and maintaining weight loss. Writing down very little of these critical aspects of weight control usually results in very minimal or temporary success. These findings are so clear and so consistent that they support the following very dramatic assertion:

> If you could maintain a written record of everything you eat and all of your exercising for the next ten years, or at least 75 percent of your eating and exercising behaviors, you would *almost certainly* become an effective weight controller.

The Benefits of Very Consistent Self-Monitoring: Research Evidence

- Among weight controllers in a twelve-week program, those who self-monitored consistently lost 64 percent more weight than the inconsistent self-monitors; the consistent self-monitors also maintained this superior weight loss three months later.
- Weight controllers who discontinued self-monitoring during a five-week holiday season (Thanksgiving to New Year's) gained fifty-seven times as much weight as their counterparts who continued to self-monitor consistently.
- Out of ten changes in eating habits that were measured, only self-monitoring was clearly related to successful weight loss when evaluated almost two years after the program began.
- Two studies showed that even weight controllers who generally self-monitored very consistently discontinued monitoring for a day or more sometimes. During the weeks that they self-monitored inconsistently, however, they lost much less weight than usual for them. More specifically, when these generally consistent self-monitors kept track of virtually everything they ate and all of their exercise, they lost between one and two pounds per week; during their least consistent weeks of self-monitoring they lost only half as much weight.

- Weight controllers who were generally inconsistent self-monitors gained an average of one pound per week during their least consistent self-monitoring weeks. They fared much better—in fact, they maintained their weight—during weeks in which they self-monitored almost every day.
- Only highly consistent self-monitors lost any weight during the holiday season (Thanksgiving to New Year's) in two different studies.
- Weight controllers who self-monitored very consistently in the first few weeks of several professional treatment programs maintained much greater weight losses, compared to inconsistent self-monitors, when evaluated one to two years after treatment began.

Let's consider an example of Bev's self-monitoring records on page 90 to show how self-monitoring helped Bev. Before looking at the example, spend a few seconds writing down what you have eaten today thus far. Try to notice both the details of what you ate and how you felt about your eating. Also describe your exercising, and note any reactions to the process of writing all of this down.

Consider how it would have affected you, if you were Bev, to write down these foods on this particular day. Bev noted that the amount of fat she consumed on May 7 (35 grams) exceeded her goal of 20 grams per day by quite a bit. The monitoring helped her stay aware of her *goal* and to use that goal to help her change. In fact, she used her failure to meet her goal as a way of renewing her *commitment* to strive toward eating less fat the next day. Another goal Bev failed to meet concerned exercise. Bev attempts to exercise every day for at least a half hour. She likes to walk and uses that as a primary means of exercise. On this day, she didn't fulfill that part of her mission.

Bev has noted that she feels more in *control* and generally in a more positive *mood* when she stays focused on her eating and exercising programs. Just the process of writing and thinking about these important aspects of her life makes her feel better about herself. She also uses self-monitoring to stay aware of certain *eating patterns* and to focus on the *details* of what she eats and under what circumstances. She has learned that in order to achieve success in weight control, "the devil is in the details."

On this particular day, she realized that she neglected to eat any fruit or vegetables. Eating such excellent forms of fiber helps keep her digestion moving along effectively and also decreases her risk of colon cancer. This is one of her weaknesses and something she consistently tries to change. The details of her eating also showed relatively minimal consumption of protein from the time she woke up until 8:00 P.M. in the evening. This lack of protein, the lack of fruits and vegetables, and the substitution primarily of carbohydrates and sweets (albeit fat-free sweets) could certainly increase her chance of eating in a less controlled way in the evening. For example, she rarely eats 500-calorie muffins with 14 fat grams. Yet on this day, with its earlier imbalances, she wound up consuming the vast majority of her fat grams after 8:00 P.M. On a more positive note, she chose turkey for her sandwich meat and clearly limited her total intake to a very modest amount until the evening.

The list on the following page summarizes the benefits of self-monitoring that Bev realized, and that you could experience by self-monitoring consistently. All of these important benefits can help you persist in your efforts over time, despite the inevitable frustrations. Resolving to focus on the details can keep you going when the scale doesn't cooperate or after you eat some high-fat foods.

Bev's Self-Monitoring Record for May 7

Date: Thursday, 5/7
Exercise: None

Time	Food	Calories	Fat Grams
7:30 A.M.	Pineapple juice	130	0.0
Noon	2 yogurt puddings	380	0.0
	8 garlic breadsticks	240	8.0
8:00 P.M.	4 small turkey sandwiches		
	(on Hawaiian buns)	600	13.0
	1 muffin	500	14.0
	Total	**1,850**	**35.0**

Why Self-Monitoring Helps

Consistent self-monitoring improves weight control by:

- Increasing your ability to use GOALS
- Improving your COMMITMENT to change
- Increasing your feeling of CONTROL
- Improving your understanding of EATING and EXERCISE PATTERNS
- Improving your information about, and focus on, the DETAILS
- Promoting a more POSITIVE MOOD

Self-Monitoring Techniques

Saint Ignatius of Loyola believed in the power of self-monitoring in the 1500s. He suggested that his followers would benefit spiritually by focusing twice per day on specific written records kept about their behaviors.

> ### Self-Monitoring:
> ### A Good Idea in 1500 and in 2000
>
> Some really good ideas have no time limit. In the sixteenth century, Saint Ignatius suggested that self-monitoring can help people improve their lives. He suggested self-monitoring twice a day, every day. A person who wishes to change himself, Saint Ignatius said,
>
>> should demand an account of himself with regard to the particular point which he has resolved to watch in order to correct himself and improve. Let him go over the single hours or periods from the time he arose to the hour and moment of the present examination, and make a mark for each time he has fallen into the particular sin or defect.
>>
>> The second day should be compared with the first, that is, the two examinations of the present day with the two of the preceding day. Let him observe if there is an improvement from one day to another. Let him compare one week with another and observe whether he has improved during the present week as compared to the preceding.

Present-day weight controllers have choices among hundreds of different methods of recording information about their eating and exercising behaviors. Every bookstore sells various weight-loss diaries. Science cannot tell you which particular format will help you self-monitor. Yet after almost thirty years of experience in helping thousands of weight controllers, I have seen many successful weight controllers use three variations of self-monitoring techniques very effectively: basic self-monitoring, condensed self-monitoring, and computerized self-monitoring.

The passages below give examples of each of these approaches. By reviewing them carefully, you can find the technique that you can use most comfortably and consistently. Remember, consistency in self-monitoring is the key. Whatever technique you use, in order for you to succeed at losing weight, you have to find an approach that you are very likely to use every single day. As suggested in the following quiz, accuracy in self-monitoring is also highly desirable.

After you achieve your weight-loss goal and have maintained it for many months, you can decrease your self-monitoring. At that point, you can simply weigh yourself on a regular basis (at least weekly) and then use self-monitoring, once again, if your weight begins to increase by a couple of pounds. In this way, self-monitoring is a tool that you can use throughout your life to increase your ability to focus very specifically on your eating and exercising patterns.

Is That an Apple You're Eating—or a Small Watermelon?

Does an apple equal an apple equal an apple? Very consistent self-monitoring, even if inaccurate, greatly improves effectiveness at weight control. But consistent *and* accurate self-monitoring is even more useful and effective. To achieve accurate self-monitoring, you need to know the details of the size of typical portions. Try taking the quiz below and see how accurately you can judge some common portion sizes.

Question 1. A medium-sized orange or apple is about the same size as:
     A. a small basketball
     B. a tennis ball
     C. a grapefruit

Question 2. A 3-ounce portion of meat is about the same size as:
     A. a videotape
     B. an audiotape cassette
     C. a deck of cards

Question 3. A 1-ounce portion of cheese is about the size of:
     A. a deck of cards

B. a 3.5-inch computer disk

C. a VW Beetle

Question 4. A teaspoon of margarine is about the same size as:

A. a compact disc

B. your nose

C. the tip of your thumb

Answers: 1. B, 2. B and C, 3. B, 4. C

Basic Self-Monitoring

Pam's story shows an example of the use of the basic self-monitoring technique. By far the most important aspect of basic self-monitoring is the recording of specific information about all foods eaten every day. Whether or not you record details, such as calories consumed and fat grams consumed, is far less important than the recording of your food intake and your exercise efforts. On the other hand, recording and totaling calories and fat grams consumed allows you to use the power of goal setting to your advantage.

Pam's Final Battle

Pam was a forty-two-year-old public relations executive when she began what she called her "final battle." Pam had many issues concerning food that had resulted in anorexia (extreme thinness due to self-starvation) as a young adult, followed by a substantial weight problem for most of her life. At the time she began her last vigorous effort to lose weight, she stood five feet, four inches tall and weighed 242 pounds.

Pam noted that her weight problem (she was approximately 100 pounds overweight) bothered her tremendously every single day of her life. Yet after trying everything that she could think of to beat it, she had given up on it in the past couple of years. That only made it worse. She was disgusted with the way she looked. Pam had enjoyed clothes very much and was a very good looking woman. She felt that this excess weight had tremendously undermined her life at work, her relationship with her husband (primarily due to her own unhappiness more than anything else), and her physical well-being. Pam was very knowledgeable about nutrition, having studied it in college. She was determined to find some way to win this final battle.

By self-monitoring very carefully, attending weekly individual therapy sessions with me, and religiously and consistently developing a treadmill and outdoor walking exercise program, Pam became very successful at weight control. She used her considerable knowledge about food and cooking to create a wide variety of interesting soups and other concoctions. Her husband was fully supportive of her efforts and actually enjoyed the change in patterns and types of foods at home. After approximately eleven months of hard work on this aspect of her life, Pam got below the 200-pound barrier. Continued efforts in the following six months brought her weight down to a much more comfortable 172 pounds. Over the past two years her weight has fluctuated between 160 and 175 pounds. Although she would like to get below 150, she found that even at 170 pounds she is able to wear very attractive clothes and has dramatically improved her self-esteem and physical well-being.

Pam exercises almost every day, often traveling as much as five miles at a time on a treadmill or walking along Chicago's lakefront. Her blood pressure has decreased, her cholesterol is lower, and she is much stronger than she has been in many years. She feels good and, compared to how she felt several years ago, is in a much better mood almost every day. She has been offered more interesting assignments at work and has had more frequent opportunities for promotion, and she believes she generally lives a more balanced life now.

Pam still struggles, however, to stay pleased and grateful (largely to herself) for what she has achieved. Part of her focuses, in a mean-spirited way, on the unfinished business of those last 20 pounds. Perhaps this edge of staying only partially satisfied with her weight-control efforts has helped her maintain the 70-pound weight loss for two years:

> I've never maintained my weight—not even for a month! When I think of that, I feel very good to look and feel and be 170 pounds instead of 240 pounds. I've got to stay positive about what I've done but avoid easing up on my approach to food or exercise. I know there's a 240-pounder in me, lurking, waiting for me to give in to extra sleep, snack on real potato chips, or say "What the hell!" in other ways. My self-monitoring is my insurance policy: It fends off that hungry 240-pounder.

Date: Friday, 3/12
Exercise: 3.5 miles (treadmill)

Time	Food	Calories	Fat Grams
Noon	2-oz. sourdough roll	200	2
	steamed carrots	50	
	3 steamed red potatoes	200	
	6 oz. broiled swordfish	300	9
7:00 P.M.	1½ cups brown rice	240	
	small baked potato	100	
	2 Tbs. fat-free sour cream	30	
	1 chicken breast	170	6
	steamed veggies	50	
10:00 P.M.	orange	100	
	½ cup fat-free yogurt	100	
	Total	**1,540**	**17**

Pam used the goal of 20 fat grams per day so that she could make adjustments in the evening, if necessary, to reach that goal every day. On some days Pam did not record the amount of fat consumed. Here's the way she compared the difference between recording and totaling fat grams versus just recording and totaling food consumed:

> Whenever I total the amount of fat grams I eat, I become much more tuned in to the little details that squeak in around the edges in my eating program. For example, at a party it's very easy to eat a little cube of cheese on a cracker. If I don't record the fat grams, which could quite easily be 5 for small cubes of cheese, I found I could talk myself into thinking it wasn't much of anything. When I get oriented to counting and focusing on every single fat gram, that's when I eliminate the cheese from that cracker and that's when I lose more weight.

It also helps to record the total amount eaten in calories, as well as recording the number of fat grams consumed. Without recording calories, you'll tend to "forget" the actual amounts of food you ate. On the other hand, people have the greatest difficulties when they discontinue self-monitoring altogether or only record some of what they eat during the day. One way of thinking about this is that perhaps 80 percent of the benefit from self-monitoring is gained from recording eating and exercising in a consistent fashion. You can gain another 20 percent of the benefit of self-monitoring by recording calories and fat consumed, an important added benefit.

Some self-monitoring formats require too much work, unless you are a particularly obsessive individual. Some of the available self-monitoring books ask you to record how you are feeling, situations that you found yourself in, and other fairly elaborate things associated with your eating and exercising patterns. Research generally supports the following acronym: KISS (Keep It Simple, Silly). The most important aspect of self-monitoring is to stay focused every day. The focusing decreases tremendously if you overburden yourself with writing out largely unnecessary details.

Condensed Self-Monitoring

Most people get the appropriate level of information and keep themselves from being overburdened by using basic self-monitoring. However, what if you reach a reasonable weight and have been self-monitoring for years? At that point, you just might benefit from a device that helps you stay a bit more aware and focused than otherwise. That is the best rationale for using condensed self-monitoring. Condensed self-monitoring provides a very quick method to keep you focused on total calories consumed per day, total fat grams consumed, and amount and consistency of exercising.

Take a look at the story below and see if you can understand why Cindy, a woman who lost 260 pounds and has maintained that loss for more than five years, chose to use condensed self-monitoring. As shown in the vignette, Cindy found it quite useful to write down simply the number of calories she consumed every day and her exercise. This type of self-monitoring takes only a few seconds per day, yet the payoff can be much better maintenance of weight loss.

Research on setting goals in business contexts shows that setting specific challenging goals improves performance by 16 percent, on average. In weight control, that might translate to someone who typically eats 1,500 calories per day managing to eat 1,260 calories per day. It also translates into exercising for 35 minutes per day instead of 30 minutes per day. These differences may not seem like much, but they add up. They can mean the difference between maintaining weight for a year versus gaining several pounds per year.

The Key to Cindy's Huge Success:
Clear Focusing and Controlled Binge Eating

Cindy lost 260 pounds! She began this odyssey at five foot two and 403 pounds. Four years later she weighed 140 pounds. Cindy reported that she had "given up" on many aspects of her life when she was so heavy. She just barely managed to go to work and survive. At this new healthy weight, she has experienced a major rebirth in her interests in music, other people, and herself.

Cindy believes some of the keys to her remarkable success include exercising every day (a brisk walk for 45 minutes), weather permitting. The only weather that doesn't permit such activity, according to Cindy, is a windchill that is twenty-five degrees below zero or even colder. Since that only happens a few times a year in Chicago, Cindy can be found walking in her neighborhood virtually every day, early in the morning before going to work.

Another critical aspect that helped Cindy lose the equivalent of two entire people is her new method of binge eating. Cindy has always had difficulties with binges. When she feels stressed or bored, for as long as she can remember, she has often eaten large quantities of food. When she weighed 400 pounds, those foods included milk shakes, french fries, cookies, and other high-fat items. Now a binge might include 10 cups of air-popped popcorn and three pears. She believes in the idea:

It's okay to deviate quantitatively, but not qualitatively.

In other words, Cindy knows that she can eat fairly large quantities of very low-fat foods without compromising her weight-control efforts. On the other hand, deviations that include eating some high-fat foods can cause rather immediate and dramatic weight gains. This occurs in part because once that barrier is broken, the tendency to eat more and other types of high-fat foods increases. Remember the potato chip company ad that said, "I bet you can't eat just one"? They were right.

Cindy has maintained her focus for many years by using a condensed form of self-monitoring. She has a little book where she writes down the number of calories she's consumed during the course of the day. For example:

Date: Tuesday, 4/1
Exercise: 45 minutes walking

150
250
200
350
200
75
50
1,275

These are some of Cindy's comments about her method of staying focused:

> I'm not sure what it is about this approach to self-monitoring that works, but it does, at least for me. I aim for 1,200 calories every day. By writing down these numbers I can see how close I'm getting. It helps me stay alert about quantities. I eat so little fat anyway that I don't find it necessary to keep track of that. So I'm mainly interested in the numbers of calories and trying to beat my goal every day.
>
> Some days I realize that I've gone over a reasonable amount by the end of lunch. By looking at these numbers, I can make a midday correction and eat a particularly light dinner.
>
> It's so easy to "forget" things you eat—especially when you wish you hadn't eaten them. I think this condensed self-monitoring keeps the details real and helps me feel in control.

You can see another variation on condensed self-monitoring in the next account. Ann found that it helped her maintain her focus and her weight when she wrote down the numbers of calories consumed in her appointment book. A somewhat technical explanation for the benefits Ann appreciated about her approach to self-monitoring concerns the Premack principle. This principle asserts that you can increase desirable behaviors by pairing those behaviors with an event that occurs frequently. In Ann's approach to condensed self-monitoring, she paired the frequent event of looking at her appointment book (something that she did at least five times per day) with a desirable behavior that she wanted to increase (focusing on her weight-control effort).

Ann's Breather

Ann was in her late thirties when we first met. She was pregnant and very concerned about eating and her weight problem. She was five feet tall and weighed 198 pounds. The pregnancy was in only its tenth week, so that Ann's weight was stable and approximately 70 pounds over where she would like it to be.

Ann had struggled with her weight most of her adult life. She was constantly trying out various diets. Three years before I met her she had given birth to her second child, and ever since then she had been gaining weight rather steadily and at what she considered to be an alarming rate. She had never been at this weight and found it extremely distressing. She prided herself on her looks, had enjoyed lots of interesting clothes when she was slimmer, and wanted to get back to a place where she could feel good about herself and the way she looked. Ann was in a business that involved many meetings with business groups, and she simply felt much more unsure about herself since this weight gain. She also found it increasingly difficult to keep up with her active young children. In addition, she wanted to feel good and be as healthy as she could during the pregnancy.

Ann began self-monitoring using the basic approach. She also focused on attempting to use her treadmill for at least 30 minutes per day and radically reduced the amount of fat she consumed (from approximately 80 fat grams per day down to 15 fat grams per day). Ann's weight stabilized with this approach, despite the growing fetus within her. However, she suffered a sad and unfortunate miscarriage approximately six weeks after beginning this effort. It took Ann approximately two weeks to recover physically and psychologically (or at least to begin recovering psychologically) after the miscarriage. She then began a weight-loss effort in earnest.

She lost weight steadily over the next six months and got to a much healthier and more comfortable weight of 158. Her exercise was fairly consistent, and she ate between 800 and 1,200 calories per day and very little fat. She kept her self-monitoring booklet religiously, only missing a few days during the entire twenty-six weeks it took her to lose 40 pounds. Ann still struggled with the exercise aspect periodically. She found it difficult to exercise in the morning, but by the time she got home she'd feel exhausted and want to spend time with her children. Fortunately, she had a very supportive husband who encouraged her and provided her with the leeway to exercise in the evenings on most days.

Ann's weight loss came to a somewhat surprising halt after the initial 40 pounds. After a few weeks, she told me that she was undergoing a variety of fertility-enhancement procedures. This focus and renewed energy spent on becoming pregnant again had decreased her interest in weight control. At the heart of it was her view that if she became pregnant (or when she became pregnant), she would no longer be able to continue losing weight anyway. It was simply too difficult for her to focus very vigorously on losing weight when she felt that biologically the effort would be modified considerably sometime relatively soon.

She and I therefore decided to meet less frequently and to alter her self-monitoring technique in accord with her desire to take a "breather" from a truly intensely focused effort at losing weight. The plan for the breather was to continue the same style of eating that had gotten her to this new and much happier state. The goal was also to maintain exercise for similar reasons. In order to increase the likelihood that that would occur, Ann decided to keep track of the calories she consumed per day in her appointment book. This process took only a few seconds, but those were a few seconds wisely used. When she wrote down what she was eating she thought about it. She thought about whether it was meeting her standards in terms of fat consumption and total calories. She thought about her goal of eating approximately 1,100 to 1,300 calories per day. She thought about why this mattered in the long run. Ann considered the fact that she had made major strides in the last four months and that she didn't want to throw that away. She also realized that if she wasn't focused when she became pregnant, she might very easily gain excessive amounts of weight.

By writing down numbers of calories consumed in her appointment book, Ann realized that she was eating less fruit and fewer vegetables than she had been in the past. This information helped her modify her eating patterns to decrease her appetite and to maintain her weight.

Monday, March 8		Calories
7:00		250
8:00		
9:00		
10:00	Staff Meeting	100
11:00		
12:00	Lunch with Joan	350
1:00		
2:00		
3:00	Charlie	
4:00		150
5:00	Michael	
6:00	Call Alice	
7:00		
8:00		450
		1,300

Condensed self-monitoring probably helped Ann maintain her weight, because she not only recorded the numbers of calories she consumed in her appointment book but she taught herself to analyze where the calories were coming from. She also considered why it was a good thing to stay focused, and how she could make each day an effective day. If Ann had just blindly written down a bunch of numbers, that would have done her no good. She had to learn how to attach some meaning to those numbers to reawaken her commitment to weight control.

Computerized Self-Monitoring

In the age of laptops, palmtops, voice-recognition software, E-mail, and related developments, computerized self-monitoring has become increasingly popular with my clients. Below are two examples of computerized self-monitoring. In the first, Arlene found it motivating to record her eating and exercising within her E-mail account at home, and also to send a copy of it to her E-mail account at work. By corresponding with herself in this way, she kept herself thinking about the importance of her weight-control effort.

Arlene: You've Got E-mail—from Yourself!

Arlene, a forty-one-year-old stockbroker and mother of two, began her most recent weight control effort at five foot six and 210 pounds. Arlene came from a tradition of relatively high-fat eating and had never followed a consistent exercise regimen. She began self-monitoring and using a basic technique (writing in a pocket-sized book). Her exercise approach emphasized everyday activities, such as walking to and from a train to get to work, as opposed to a more formal and consistent routine every morning. That was one of her weaknesses as a weight controller. In addition, her heritage of high-fat eating was difficult to leave behind, and this intensive method of weight control required that she do so almost completely. After some major changes in her job and her husband's job, she found herself regaining some of the 60 pounds that she had lost in two years.

When Arlene's weight started approaching 200 pounds again, she decided she had to find a way to self-monitor that could help her maintain her interest. As someone who was very familiar with computers, she created a self-monitoring technique. She began self-monitoring using her E-mail at home. Then she forwarded the records she kept at the end of every day to her work E-mail address. As soon as she got to work she was reminded by her computer: "You've got mail!" This got her to take a look at her records on a regular basis. She just kept sending herself messages back and forth about her eating and exercising patterns.

The initial enthusiasm for this new E-mail self-monitoring technique helped Arlene relose about 10 pounds. Some vacationing interrupted this approach, however. That's one of its disadvantages. Many people do not want to take their laptops with them when they go on vacations or travel. Arlene had become somewhat dependent on this vehicle as a means for self-monitoring. Of course, she could have always resorted to a basic self-monitoring approach while traveling. But being a mere mortal, she didn't do that. She regained some of the initial 10 pounds that she had lost. Once her normal routine returned, however, so did her E-mail self-monitoring. Arlene got her weight to the low 170s again after a few additional months of hard labor.

Date: 10/20, Tuesday
20 min. gym; walking to and from the train; 8 blks. walk
Weight: 171

6:30	milk in coffee	20/0
	2 saltines w/ham	60/0.5
7:30	milk in coffee	20/0
1:00	veggie burrito	300/5
	instant soup	80/3.5

5:00	fat-free Olestra chips	75/0
6:00	strawberry fat-free shake	70/0
7:00	slice of bread	70/1
8:00	stuffed egg white with fat-free	
	sour cream and mustard	50/0
	broiled swordfish	260/8.8
	boiled ½ potato	80/0
	skim latte	50/0
11:00	boiled egg white	20/0
		1,155/18.8

Karl's method involves a somewhat more traditional use of the computer. Karl is a computer specialist (a software consultant). He has a computer with him at almost all times and finds it very easy to use existing software programs to analyze his self-monitoring data. These nutritional software programs automatically total calories and fat eaten by the end of each day and summarize this information at the end of each week. Many of these programs also provide color graphics to show patterns over days, weeks, and months. The disadvantage of this approach is that it requires fluency with typing, tolerance for some missing information in the software programs, and a willingness to put some extra time into self-monitoring.

Karl's Self-Monitoring via Software

Karl's 402 pounds began taking a very major toll on his life and well-being, even at the relatively young age of thirty-four.

His five-foot-ten frame simply couldn't support that amount of weight. When I met him he had already undergone a series of hospitalizations for problems with circulation in his legs. He'd also started having increasing difficulties walking and keeping up with his two young children. Karl also maintained his own small computer software consultation business. His health problems interfered with his vitality and his eagerness to develop the business to its full potential.

Karl used his substantial skills with computers and with software to self-monitor. Through consistent self-monitoring, major changes in the fat content of his eating, and the beginnings of a walking program, Karl lost nearly 75 pounds in just six months. At the time of this writing, he showed no signs of decelerating these efforts.

One of the things Karl noticed through his very diligent and complete self-monitoring was that in the weeks where his total fat intake averaged above 20 fat grams, his rate of weight loss declined considerably. In contrast, when his fat consumption averaged closer to 10 grams per day, his rate of weight loss seemed to double. Take a look at the following two examples of Karl's self-monitoring data generated on a software program. The first example certainly shows relatively low-fat eating; but the second example shows the more extreme low-fat eating advocated in this book. The latter style of eating was the one associated with his more dramatic weight loss.

A Somewhat-Higher-Fat-Intake Day

2/11	*Calories*	*Fat*
Exercise: 25 min. swinging golf clubs; 25-min. walk		
1 muffin, no fat	150.00	0.00
1 milk, no fat	90.00	0.00
2 milk, no fat	180.00	0.00
2 hot dog, no fat	90.00	0.00
2 bread, wheat	130.00	2.05
1 bag chips	75.00	0.00
1 cookie, no fat, oatmeal raisin	100.00	0.00
.5 cup beans, green, butter sauce	30.00	1.00
.5 cup rice and sauce, long grain	121.30	0.20

2/11	*Calories*	*Fat*
1 chicken, breast, no skin, roasted	85.80	1.86
1 chicken, thigh, no skin, roasted	64.79	3.37
1 chicken, wing, with skin, roasted	60.90	4.09
1 chicken, leg, with skin, roasted	160.10	9.29
2 milk, no fat	180.00	0.00
1 cake, carrot	170.00	5.00
2 milk, no fat	180.00	0.00
.5 cup ice cream, fat free, chc/vn	100.00	0.00
Total for 02/11	**1,967.89**	**26.86**

A Low-Fat-Intake Day

02/17	*Calories*	*Fat*
Diary Contents		
Exercise: 4 15-min. walks, bowling		
1 muffin, no fat	150.00	0.00
1 milk, no fat	90.00	0.00
2 bread, wheat	130.00	2.05
2 turkey, breast, slices	81.00	1.42
1 lettuce, iceberg, raw	2.60	0.04
1 tomato, red, ripe, raw	25.83	0.41
1 bag chips, baked	130.00	1.50
3 milk, no fat	270.00	0.00
3 bread, wheat	195.00	3.07
2 hot dog, no fat	90.00	0.00
3 bologna, fat free	210.00	0.00
1 bag chips	90.00	1.00
8 oz. soup, chicken broth, no fat	39.04	0.00
.25 chicken, breast, no skin, stewed	21.52	0.43

02/17	*Calories*	*Fat*
.25 cup Mushrooms, Boiled	0.81	0.01
.3 oz. pasta, fresh, ckd	11.14	0.09
1 tbsp onion, boiled	6.60	0.03
.3 garlic, raw	1.34	0.00
.5 cup ice cream, fat free, chc/vn	100.00	0.00
1 milk, no fat	90.00	0.00
Total	**1,734.88**	**10.05**

Every diet encourages you to decrease your eating and change the type of eating that you do. Diets also attempt to give you hope, help you focus on this issue in your life, and, perhaps most importantly, help you increase your awareness about eating and exercising. The helpful aspects of any diet lie in these factors, not in the magic of grapefruit or the latest ideas in combining foods. The scientific approach that I advocate cuts directly to the chase and provides a method of staying very clearly aware of your eating and exercising patterns every day and every week. This awareness tells you the single most important concept in self-monitoring:

Everything counts!

Weight control does not begin on a Monday or on the first day of a new month or on the first day of a new year. It begins as soon as you can stay focused and make a sincere effort to control your eating and exercising. By self-monitoring very consistently, you learn that even if you start the day with bacon and eggs, you can finish the day with low-fat eating. Bacon and eggs do not contain an infinite number of calories or fat grams. You can count the fat grams in any food and realize that you can neutralize the effects of whatever problem food you consumed by eating more effectively at your next opportunity. Self-monitoring can help you do that. *If you cannot live with the notion that everything counts, you will not succeed at weight control.*

Self-monitoring can take many forms. Regardless of the form it takes, it must include some written record of your eating and exercising that covers every day. It should also include a record of your weight. If you know how much you are eating and exercising and you know your weight at any given point in time, you are staying in the struggle to succeed. If you give up this knowledge, you allow your biology to take over. Whether you monitor via computer or use some condensed version of self-monitoring, *you can find a way to succeed if you can find a way to stay aware of the details.*

F I V E

❖

Exercising Enough

Truth #7: Exercise every day is the way.

Steve's Long Climb to Success

Steve Silva's tears of joy told the story. The ordeal was over. Steve had just completed his heroic assault on the world record for the vertical mile. He had raced up and down the Eiffel Tower seven and a half times, covering a heart-thumping 9,127 steps in 2 hours, 2 minutes, and 54 seconds.

Steve had finished just 1½ minutes shy of the world record. "I wasn't crying because I didn't make it," said a smiling Silva a few minutes later. "I was just so glad to finish!" By finishing, Steve Silva had achieved a much longer climb than the Eiffel Tower race. Eight years prior to that moment, Steve had weighed 435 pounds. A thirty-nine-year-old high school teacher, he had lost 100 pounds six different times, only to gain it all, and more, back each time. Steve had ankle problems that made jogging and some other forms of exercise impossible, so he'd decided to climb stairs. He'd lost 245 pounds (down to a trim and powerful 190 pounds) by climbing up and down 30,000 steps a week.

Steve's weight still fluctuates, but now, he says, "I eat more, but more veggies. I've learned to have more undereating weeks than overeating weeks." He advises others, "Make some reasonable changes; don't expect miracles." This is good advice from a man who has had more experience than almost anyone with life's ups and downs.

Exercise Facts and Fictions

How much do you know about exercising? Most weight controllers accept its importance, but confusions about it are very common. Please take the following test to evaluate the status of your current knowledge.

Exercise Test

Circle the best answer for each question.

1. Exercise doesn't promote weight loss as much as most people think; it takes a lot of exercise to burn off a few calories.   *True*   *False*

2. Sit-ups can help you lose fat from the midsection of your body.   *True*   *False*

3. Swimming does not help people lose weight.   *True*   *False*

4. Overweight people do not have underactive metabolisms.   *True*   *False*

5. Increasing daily activities (such as climbing more stairs and walking farther from parking places) does not help people lose weight.   *True*   *False*

6. Running three miles burns the same number of calories as walking those three miles.   *True*   *False*

7. Women and men burn the same number of calories when they do the same activities.   *True*   *False*

8. Jogging five miles per day every day of the week is the ideal exercise regimen for most people.	*True*	*False*
9. Exercise can increase appetite.	*True*	*False*
10. Exercise cannot affect bones and posture.	*True*	*False*
11. If you exercise at the level of your maximum heart rate for more than five minutes, you may die.	*True*	*False*
12. It is impossible to maintain the same level of cardiovascular fitness in your sixties that you had when you were in your twenties.	*True*	*False*
13. Weight lifting is appropriate for people under fifty, but it presents many risks, especially for those who are older.	*True*	*False*
14. Exercising can improve cholesterol levels.	*True*	*False*
15. Exercise can improve resting metabolic rate.	*True*	*False*

Answers and Explanations

1. *False*

Exercise does promote weight loss at least as much as most people think. First, you expend significant amounts of calories during the exercise itself. For example, a fast walk for about 40 minutes burns off 200 calories. Second, you expend calories after the walk stops. That is, to replenish the energy consumed during exercise, the body must work harder than it does when it is resting. This increases your metabolism.

Metabolism is the energy expended by the body to maintain itself (for example, through breathing, digestion, and excretion). Metabolism (or metabolic rate) may remain higher than normal for up to twenty-four hours after exercising. This means that the energy expended by exercising may increase substantially throughout the rest of the day after the exercise is completed. This increase in energy expenditure may amount to doubling the initial amount of calories burned off during the exercise.

Third, energy expended during the exercise and by elevating metabolism accumulates day by day, week by week. For example, the 40-minute fast walk, if completed every day, may amount to as much as one pound lost per week. That's 50 pounds per year. Fourth, exercising helps reinforce your commitment to weight control. When you exercise, you might think, "Why am I out here sweating when I could be home sleeping?" You may then remind yourself, "I'm out here because I want to control my weight, to look good, to be healthy. I'm here because I'm taking charge of this thing."

2. *False*
Sit-ups cannot help you lose fat from your stomach (midsection).

"Spot reduction" simply does not work. Your body takes fat supplies from places that it is directed to by your hormones and genetics. However, sit-ups can improve muscle tone. This could allow you to improve your posture and the appearance of your midsection. You can do this without consciously holding in your stomach. In addition, the improvement in muscle tone from sit-ups and related crunches can decrease back problems. When you improve muscle tone in the front and sides of your body, you place less pressure on your back (particularly your lower back). Since 80 to 90 percent of adult Americans develop some back problems (and even a higher percentage of obese people develop these problems), the benefits of sit-ups and crunches are clear.

3. *False*
Swimming can help people lose weight. A recent study received a lot of attention because it seemed to show that swimming did not help people lose weight. However, this study was flawed; there are many

other ways of explaining the results. The biological reality is that any energy expenditure can help you lose weight. Swimming places very little strain on the back, the knees, and other weak parts of the body. If you swim approximately 20 yards per minute, you will expend approximately 100 calories in about 25 minutes. If you sit down for 25 minutes, you'll expend approximately 25 calories—that is, about 25 percent of the calories burned when swimming at that slow pace. If you swim at 50 yards per minute, for example, you'll expend 100 calories in about 8 minutes. That's about twelve times more calories burned than by sitting.

4. *False*

Some overweight people do have underactive metabolisms. Metabolic rates vary just as all biological functions do. Some people are very efficient and expend relatively few calories to keep themselves functioning. Other people are much more inefficient and expend far more calories to keep themselves breathing, digesting, and staying alive. Exercise can increase metabolic rates.

5. *False*

Increasing daily activities (such as climbing more stairs and parking farther from stores, thereby causing more walking) can help you lose weight. Any expenditure of energy can help promote weight loss. When you expend more energy than you take in, you lose weight. You expend energy every minute of your life. If you are sitting down or watching television, you expend about one calorie per minute. As soon as you stand up, you burn two calories per minute. When you start moving around a little bit, you burn three calories per minute. If you start running, energy expenditure may go up to ten calories or more per minute. Recently one of my newer clients came to a session eager to report on her increase in exercise. She had joined an aerobics class and had begun going to it three times per week. She also discussed her other activities. It turns out she had also started gardening recently. She spent a few minutes calculating the number of calories expended during a recent weekend's gardening.

She gardened for approximately four hours on both Saturday and Sunday of that weekend. Based on her weight and the calories expended per minute in those activities, calculations showed that she burned approximately 1,200 calories per day by gardening on both Saturday and Sunday. In contrast, her low-impact aerobics class probably resulted in an expenditure of only 300 calories per class. This means that one afternoon's gardening accounted for greater expenditure of energy than all three aerobics classes in that week! She was amazed. She had lost three pounds that week and had attributed that substantial weight loss to the aerobics classes. Her gardening actually accounted for much more of the weight loss than did the aerobics classes. The lesson here is that whenever you have the opportunity to exercise, even informally, take it.

6. *True*

Running three miles does burn approximately the same number of calories as walking those three miles. For example, when a 154-pound man runs at an 8-minute-mile pace, he will expend 100 calories in approximately 7 minutes. If that same man walks at a 17-minute-mile pace, he will expend the same 100 calories in approximately 14 minutes. This man could walk the first mile in about 17 minutes and then run the second mile in about 8 minutes (25 minutes total). If he did this, he would expend approximately 200 calories. He could also walk those two miles in 34 minutes and burn the same 200 calories.

Running provides the advantages of expending energy in a lot less time, and it may produce a longer-lasting increase in metabolic rate for several hours or so. Walking has the advantage of being less painful to do. Walking also produces fewer injuries to knees and backs than running does. I have had quite a few clients who lost a lot of weight using running as their primary exercise. I have had many more clients lose weight using walking as their primary exercise. For example, one of my clients lost 250 pounds doing no other exercise than fast walking (approximately 40 minutes per day).

7. *False*
Since most men weigh considerably more than most women, women and men usually do not burn the same number of calories when they do the same activities. If a man and a woman weighed the same amount, they would burn approximately the same number of calories doing the same activities. For example, a 154-pound person would take 10 minutes to expend 100 calories when running a 12-minute mile. A 128-pound person would take 12 minutes, running at that same pace, to burn 100 calories.

8. *False*
Jogging five miles per day every day of the week is not the ideal exercise regimen for most people. Jogging is a wonderful form of exercise. It is efficient and it produces many benefits. However, jogging pounds the knees, jars the hips, crunches the spinal column, and can contribute to a variety of back problems. The risk of knee, back, hip, and other problems increases substantially if you jog more than five days per week. These orthopedic risks also increase substantially when you jog for more than 30 minutes per outing. Since almost everyone would take quite a bit more than 30 minutes to jog five miles, the combination of jogging five miles plus jogging seven out of seven days creates a substantial risk for injury.

Overweight people in particular would be ill advised to attempt such a regimen. Excess weight creates excess pounding on the knees and increases the likelihood of foot, hip, and back problems. Walking seven days per week, on the other hand, would create few such problems.

9. *True*

Exercise can increase appetite; but mild to moderate exercise can actually decrease *appetite.* For example, most people find they desire food less if they exercise 10, 15, 20, or even 60 minutes. However, exercising for several hours often *increases* appetite. You can prevent this increase in appetite by eating or drinking beverages with calories during extended periods of exercise. Liquids are easiest to digest during exercise, and carbohydrates are also relatively easy to digest. For example, fruit juices and fruit make good appetite suppressants during extended exercise.

10. *False*

Exercise can affect bones and posture. After about age thirty-five, a person's bone mass (sometimes called bone density) gradually decreases. This bone loss can lead to osteoporosis, the weakening of your bones—causing them to break easily. Exercise preserves bone mass.

Consider what happens when adults stay in bed (for example, during illness or hospitalization). They typically lose as much bone mass in two weeks as they would normally lose in a year. Studies have shown that exercising regularly can actually build bone in older people. One such study showed an increase in bone mass in a group of women whose average age was eighty-one.

11. *False*

You can exercise at the level of your maximum heart rate for far more than five minutes without any concern about dying. You could actually survive at your maximum heart rate for many days. This principle holds unless you have a heart condition.

12. *False*

It is very possible to maintain the same level of cardiovascular fitness in your sixties that you had when you were in your twenties. Remember your hunter-gatherer ancestry. Hunter-gatherers maintained high levels of activity throughout their lifetimes. People in industrialized countries maintain high levels of activity during childhood (at least most people do), but they become more and more sedentary as they get older. Inactivity begets weakness; weakness begets injuries and more weakness. Studies show that regular aerobic exercise can maintain cardiovascular fitness and can even reverse some of the damage done by sedentary living. For example, in a recent study, nineteen men and women in their sixties exercised aerobically for about one hour three times per week. After two months, their resting metabolic rates increased by about 10 percent (on average), virtually eliminating the decline in resting metabolic rate caused naturally by the aging process.

Aerobic capacities, or fitness levels, can also improve radically with persistent exercising. Many reports testify to the remarkable conditioning of runners and other committed athletes who were measured in their youth and then again in old age. Very few declines in aerobic conditioning occurred for these athletes. As people grow older, reflexes slow down and some decreases in flexibility seem almost inevitable. But cardiovascular fitness can be maintained at very high levels. Sixty-year-olds can, indeed, have cardiovascular systems like twenty-year-olds. The table on pages 120 to 124 documents this point quite dramatically.

13. *False*
Weight lifting is very appropriate for people of all ages. With proper supervision, even ninety-year-olds can benefit from weight lifting. For example, a study with ten ninety-year-olds had them lift weights with their legs for 10 to 20 minutes, three times per week. After eight weeks, they could lift three times more weight than they could prior to beginning weight lifting. Two of the nonagenarians gave up their canes after just eight weeks of lifting.

14. *True*

Exercise can improve cholesterol levels. Some evidence suggests that regular exercising can increase the level of HDL, or "good cholesterol."

15. *True*

Exercise can improve resting metabolic rate. Metabolic rate refers to the rate at which your body uses (metabolizes) energy when you are resting. Your body uses quite a bit of energy even when you are resting in order to digest food, keep you breathing, and so on. Studies with both animals and humans show that your body slows down your metabolic rate when you start eating less than usual. This would allow you to survive during food shortages, when the hunting and gathering is not going well. If you exercise regularly, however, your body reacts as if everything is okay. If you are moving around a lot, then your body "knows" you must not be starving. So every day that you exercise, your body will keep your metabolic rate high. This important effect means that on days that you exercise, your body will expend more energy all day, thus allowing you to lose weight more easily than if you hadn't exercised that day.

The Benefits of Exercising

This test makes it clear that exercising is critical for effective weight control. Steven Blair also made this point with a quiz published in 1991 in the *Weight Control Digest*. You may improve your commitment to exercising if you understand the many ways exercise can affect you. While you know exercise can improve your ability to control your weight, do you know how exercising can affect you as you grow older? The comparisons below show critical differences between the fit person you can become versus the sedentary person that you must stop being in order to succeed. Fitness provides increasing and more dramatic benefits as you get older.

Only the Fit Stay Young:
Changes in Women's Bodies
at 20, 30, 40, 50, 60, and 70*

TWENTIES

The Fit Woman

. . . she retains the strength, stamina and flexibility of her teen years. Her leanness allows the definition of her muscles to show through. Late in this decade her bone strength may reach its peak. If she continues regular weight-bearing exercises, consumes plenty of calcium-rich foods and gets adequate caloric intake, her bones will stay healthy for years to come. A lot of time spent outdoors without adequate sun protection will cause her skin to begin to freckle and develop very fine lines.

The Sedentary Woman

. . . she may look great, but physical changes are already beginning to take place that could have far-reaching effects. Her aerobic capacity begins to decline at the rate of 1 percent per year. After age 25, muscle mass can decrease by an average of 5 percent every decade. Metabolism begins to drop at a rate of 2 percent per year, which will translate into increasingly higher body-fat percentages. Any fat added now will be distributed evenly throughout her body. She will begin to experience tightness in her hips.

*Reprinted, with permission, from *Self* magazine, September 1992.

THIRTIES

The Fit Woman

. . . she looks and feels as fit as in her twenties. She's agile and coordinated, with a lean, defined physique, thanks to well-developed muscles and below-average body fat, and her aerobic capacity—the ability to transport oxygen throughout the body—is better than ever. She will, however, begin to experience an unavoidable decline in the number of fast-twitch muscles, which are responsible for quick reaction time and for high-intensity activities like sprinting. If bone strength has not yet peaked, it will by age 35.

The Sedentary Woman

. . . she will begin to feel her age in terms of muscle strength, particularly in her arms and legs. This is because her muscle fibers are starting to atrophy, and her muscle mass will continue to decline at a rate of about 6.6 percent each decade from here on out. She feels stiffer, as elastin is lost from her muscles. She could have as much as 33 percent body fat, most of it concentrated in her hips and thighs. Along with that of her active peers, her sexual responsiveness reaches a peak—but she may not have the energy to enjoy it.

FORTIES

The Fit Woman

. . . she remains as energetic and flexible as ever, with excellent aerobic stamina. Because of an inevitable decline in metabolism, however, she may have a tendency to put on some fat—particularly in her hips and

The Sedentary Woman

. . . she is by now 15 percent weaker than she was in her thirties, and the decline will be even more dramatic past age 45. Her shoulders appear narrower as muscle mass decreases in her upper back. The disks between

FORTIES *(continued)*

thighs. But her high ratio of muscle to fat keeps her calorie-burning capacity up, and this, along with continued aerobic exercise, will counteract this tendency, keeping her at about 22 percent body fat. Although she experiences some compression of the vertebrae in her back, strong muscles keep her stomach relatively flat, her back supple.

her vertebrae begin to compress, so that with time she will be 1 to 1½ inches shorter, and her stomach will distend as the distance between her ribs and pelvis decreases. She has lost about 40 percent of the range of motion in her hips and may develop varicose veins.

FIFTIES

The Fit Woman

. . . she has maintained every aspect of fitness. Her age shows only in her percentage of body fat, which continues to increase slightly—it's probably up to about 24 percent now. Gravity may start to take its toll on her body, and she may feel some wear and tear in her joints due to years of activity. She may want to rethink her workouts, switching to lower-impact activity—swimming or walking, for example.

The Sedentary Woman

. . . she has poor posture due to the continued drop in flexibility and muscle strength. She slouches forward, and has a protruding stomach and overarched lower back. All the repercussions of inadequate aerobic activity begin to kick in: Her blood pressure rises; she becomes more susceptible to diabetes and heart attacks. Now body fat begins to settle around her middle, her skin wrinkles and is tugged downward by gravity.

SIXTIES

The Fit Woman

. . . she has strong, flexible muscles and plenty of stamina. Despite the effect menopause has on estrogen production, her bones are strong thanks in part to the weight-bearing exercises and strength training she's done all her life (although hormone replacement may be necessary). Her target heart rate will be about 115 beats per minute (down 30 or 40 bpm from her twenties). But because aerobic exercise has kept her heart strong, she remains able to pump healthy amounts of blood. She has about 26 percent body fat.

The Sedentary Woman

. . . she is two or three inches shorter by now and may have developed osteoporosis, partly because she has not done the weight-bearing exercise that keeps bones strong. Her breasts begin to sag in earnest and her waist widens even more. Her heart is 10 to 15 percent weaker than it was when she was 20, and measurable changes in her immune system increase her risk of developing cancer and certain infections. Wrinkles are now creases, and skin is dry.

SEVENTIES

The Fit Woman

. . . she can work and play almost as hard as she did 30 years ago. Only a slight increase in body fat—amplified by the earth's pull—reveals her age, along with deeper creases in her face and a drier look to her skin due to a decline in oil

The Sedentary Woman

. . . she is in failing health as high blood pressure, brittle bones and unhealthy blood cholesterol levels leave her vulnerable to a host of serious diseases. Her flexibility, strength and stamina are about nil, and she may have developed the

SEVENTIES *(continued)*

production that occurs after menopause.

classic "dowager's hump." She has wrinkles in her cheeks, and her mouth turns down, so she appears as unhappy as she probably feels.

The exercise test and the comparison of fit versus sedentary women show many benefits of exercising. The following list describes even more.

Exercise can:

1. Increase weight loss
2. Improve maintenance of weight losses
3. Improve stress management
4. Improve the quality of sleep
5. Improve digestion
6. Enhance self-esteem
7. Improve resistance to illnesses
8. Help you feel energized
9. Promote better digestion and bowel functioning
10. Tone muscles
11. Provide more definition to muscles
12. Reduce blood pressure
13. Reduce tension
14. Improve flexibility
15. Build strength
16. Promote greater endurance
17. Decrease the negative effects of aging
18. Decrease menstrual cramping
19. Increase metabolic rate
20. Enhance coordination

21. Improve posture
22. Decrease back problems and pain
23. Decrease resting heart rate
24. Strengthen bones and joints
25. Improve reaction time
26. Strengthen the heart
27. Prevent heart disease
28. Improve cholesterol levels
29. Prevent osteoporosis (weakness of the bones)
30. Decrease the risk of cancer (particularly colon cancers)
31. Improve ability to relax more quickly
32. Decrease depression
33. Increase emotional stability
34. Improve quality of thinking
35. Improve ability to stay warm in colder climates
36. Improve ability to tolerate warmer climates
37. Improve agility
38. Improve body image
39. Increase endorphins (internally produced opiates that improve feelings of well-being and positive mood)
40. Decrease constipation
41. Improve social life (for example, you can meet new people during exercising)
42. Improve athletic performance
43. Increase life span
44. Increase feelings of control or mastery
45. Improve rosiness of complexion
46. Decrease appetite
47. Provide balance in life
48. Increase self-awareness
49. Provide time to think, gain perspective, and solve problems more effectively
50. Promote self-actualization

This is a rather convincing list, isn't it? Many of the benefits of exercise pertain directly to weight control. Changes in muscles, bones, fat, and attitude can all affect success at weight control. In fact, some studies of successful weight controllers show that virtually 100 percent of successful weight controllers become frequent exercisers. Some of these studies included people who lost 50 pounds or more and maintained the loss for more than five years. On average, these master weight controllers walk briskly for one hour per day— every day. Only 20 percent of Americans over twenty-five years old exercise at least twice per week. This also means that most Americans—the sedentary ones—place themselves at unnecessarily high risk for developing cancer, as described below.

Can Exercise Prevent Cancer?

Seventy years ago, two Minnesota physicians noticed that most of their patients who developed cancer led sedentary lives. They also noticed that patients who were farmers rarely developed cancer. They speculated that hard work and physical activity might prevent cancer. They compared cancer rates among various occupations. As they expected, cancer rates decreased as physical activity increased.

More recent research has supported the idea that exercising regularly can prevent cancer. A study of thirteen thousand people conducted by the Institute for Aerobics Research in Dallas used the treadmill test to measure fitness levels and then track cancer rates over eight years. They found that the men who were least fit had more than four times the overall cancer rates than the most fit men. The least fit women had sixteen times higher death rates due to cancer than the most fit women.

Many studies show that exercising decreases risks of colon cancer, breast cancer, and possibly prostate cancer. Cancer of the colon is the second leading cause of death (next to lung cancer) in the United States. Fifty thousand Americans die each year from this type of cancer. Twenty-one of twenty-seven recent studies have found that as activity increases, rates of colon cancer decrease.

Exercise may prevent colon cancer by increasing the speed at which waste products get through the colon. Greater physical activity leads to greater mobility in the intestines, as well. Also, greater physical activity might affect some biochemical agents that promote increased speed of digestion. It follows that the less time waste products spend in the colon, the less time those waste products that contain cancer-causing substances (carcinogens) spend in the body.

An important study on breast cancer involved more than five thousand women who graduated from college between 1925 and 1981. The women who had been college athletes had about half the risk of breast cancer as the nonathletes. Another study of twenty-five thousand women in the state of Washington showed that those who had worked in physically active jobs had much lower incidences of breast cancer than those who had sedentary occupations. Exercising may prevent breast cancer because it lowers estrogen levels.

Research on more than seventeen thousand Harvard alumni showed that among men over age seventy, those who had remained most active had much lower incidences of prostate cancer than the least active men. However, the "most active" men expended more than 3,000 calories per week in walking, climbing stairs, and playing sports compared to the least active men. It takes a lot of activity to expend 3,000 calories. High levels of activity may decrease levels of the male hormone testosterone. Lowering this hormone may decrease the risk of prostate cancer.

Frequent exercisers tend to have other habits associated with the decreased risk of cancer. For example, frequent exercisers smoke less and eat lower-fat diets than sedentary people. However, most of the studies on exercise and cancer did eliminate these factors when analyzing the effects of exercise. In other words, those studies found that exercising reduces risks of getting cancer regardless of the effects of diet and smoking. It seems safe to conclude that exercising regularly can prevent cancer.

How to Exercise to Lose Weight

Is it advisable to exercise every day? Is it advisable to exercise for 20 minutes per day? Or 40, 60, 120? What kind of exercising produces optimal results for weight controllers: aerobic exercise, weight lifting, or a combination of both? Do everyday activities like walking to a bus or shopping help people lose weight?

The American College of Sports Medicine (ACSM) has provided recommendations to answer these questions. ACSM consists of many of the world's premier experts on exercising. Their most recent set of recommendations has become accepted around the world as the basis for developing safe and effective exercising patterns. Let's review answers to commonly asked questions by considering five aspects of exercising and the ACSM recommendations that pertain to them:

- Frequency of exercise
- Intensity of exercise
- Duration of exercise
- Mode of exercise
- Strength training (weight lifting)

Frequency of Exercise

Since exercising is so critical to weight control, I strongly encourage each of my clients to exercise every single day. This exercise can vary from walking to swimming to playing racquetball. If you become accustomed to exercising in some form every day, you will lose more weight and maintain that weight loss more effectively.

This recommendation of seven days per week is somewhat unusual. ACSM recommends four to six days per week to maintain a good level of fitness. However, because of the many benefits for weight control, I recommend placing an even greater emphasis on exercise.

Setting a daily goal for exercising may well improve your consistency. People who set a permanent, daily goal may not use as many excuses to avoid exercising. If you adopted a five-day-per-week goal, you could say to yourself, "Today is the day I won't exercise. I'll exercise tomorrow." This kind of thinking allows for many reasons to skip days. Have you said to yourself, "I don't feel like it today," or "I don't have time today?" If you commit thoroughly to a daily goal, it makes it more difficult to allow yourself to postpone this critical aspect of your well-being. Some of my clients have used an expression to capture this: "Not exercising is not an option." Remember, you are pursuing something other than a general improvement in your health. You are combating biological forces that are dead set against weight loss. This takes extraordinary effort and commitment.

Intensity of Exercise

Intensity refers to how hard your body works during a certain length of time. More intensive exercise means that your body works harder for the 15 or 30 or 45 minutes during which you exercise. Intensity varies depending on your level of conditioning or fitness. For example, world-class marathoners can run three 8-minute miles in a row and barely break a sweat. To the average person, this intensity of running would prove extremely challenging. For the nonrunner's body, this intensity level would be very high. For the world-class marathoner, this intensity is very low.

Intensity of exercise is measured in several ways. The simplest way to measure it involves heart rate. The average heart rate of a forty-five-year-old man at rest is about 72 beats per minute. During moderate exercise, this increases to 145 beats per minute. Maximum exercise may lead to a heart rate of 175 beats per minute. This man's heart generally pumps about five and a half quarts of blood per minute while he is resting. During heavy exercise, his heart pumps about four times that amount of blood (22 quarts). His breathing rate goes from 12 breaths per minute to 43 breaths per minute. His systolic blood pressure goes from 120 to 200 (mmHg). These biological changes occur because the body consumes a lot of energy and a lot of oxygen when it works hard. The muscle cells consume energy in the form of stored sugar (glycogen, glucose) as well as fats. The consumption of this energy requires oxygen, which is also used quickly during intensive exercise.

Your heart has a maximum capability for pumping blood and helping your body function during intensive exercising. You can actually sustain your maximum heart rate for many hours, and even many days. However, this maximum rate is considered an upper limit from which you can judge the intensity of your exercising. Subtract your age from 220 to calculate your maximum heart rate. If you are forty years old, your maximum heart rate is 180 beats per minute ($220 - 40 = 180$). When you exercise at high-intensity levels (close to your maximum heart rate), you become exhausted very quickly. You also increase your risk of injury through sprains and strains. In contrast, when you exercise at 60 to 80 percent of your maximum heart rate (your "training heart rate"), you stress your system in a positive way. This level of overloading your cardio-vascular system can actually increase your heart's ability to pump blood throughout your body. By exercising at this recommended training heart rate, your muscles become increasingly efficient at extracting oxygen from your blood. This increase in efficiency takes time. It usually takes several weeks of fairly frequent exercise to improve efficiency at extracting oxygen from the blood and strengthening your heart. Gradually, however, anyone who exercises at this training rate enough becomes an increasingly fit individual.

Sometimes the term "aerobic capacity" is used to describe this type of fitness. "Aerobic" simply means involving oxygen. When you become aerobically fit, you increase your heart's ability to pump oxygenated blood through your body, and you increase the efficiency of your muscles at extracting oxygen from your blood. The more fit you are, the more oxygen and fuel (glucose, fat) you can get into your muscles quickly. This allows your muscles to work hard for long periods of time without producing feelings of exhaustion.

The most important rule of thumb about intensity of exercise is: *Keep the intensity low enough to allow yourself to exercise for at least 30 minutes per session*. Many people, like the birthday boy in the account below, make the mistake of exercising too intensely for their current fitness levels. As a result, they become tired and find exercise painful after only a few minutes. If you jog at a slow pace (12-minute miles), you expend about 10 calories per minute. If you walk at a moderate pace (20-minute miles), you expend about 5 calories per minute. Weight control depends on total amount of energy expended. If you can jog for only 5 minutes at the 12-minute-per-mile pace, you'll expend only 50 calories during that exercise session. On the other hand, if you can walk for 30 minutes at the moderate 20-minute-mile pace, you'll expend 150 calories. You'll expend three times more energy by exercising at the lower-intensity level. That's all that matters for weight control. *Expend energy using an intensity that you can tolerate.*

Which Is Better: Exercise or Getting Your Teeth Drilled?

For my birthday this year my wife bought me a week of private lessons at the local health club. Though still in great shape from when I was on the varsity chess team in high school, I decided it was a good idea to go ahead and try it. I called and made reservations with someone named Tanya, who said she was a twenty-six-year-old aerobics instructor and athletic clothing model. My wife seemed very pleased with how enthusiastic I was about getting started.

Day 1

They suggest I keep this "exercise diary" to chart my progress this week. Started the morning at 6:00 A.M. Tough to get up, but worth it when I arrived at the health club and Tanya was waiting for me. She's something of a goddess, with blond hair and a dazzling white smile. She showed me the machines and took my pulse after five minutes on the treadmill. She seemed a little alarmed that it was so high, but I think just standing next to her in that outfit of hers added about ten points. Enjoyed watching the aerobics class. Tanya was very encouraging as I did my sit-ups, though my gut was already aching a little from holding it in the whole time I was talking to her. This is going to be *great*.

Day 2

Took a whole pot of coffee to get me out the door, but I made it. Tanya had me lie on my back and push this heavy iron bar up into the air. Then she put weights on it, for heaven's sake! Legs were a little wobbly on the treadmill, but I made it the full mile. Her smile made it all worth it. Muscles feel *great*.

Day 3

The only way I can brush my teeth is by laying the tooth brush on the counter and moving my mouth back and forth over it. I am certain that I have developed a hernia in both pectorals. Driving was okay as long as I didn't try to steer. I parked on top of a Volkswagen. Tanya was a little impatient with me and said my screaming was bothering the other club members. The treadmill hurt my chest, so I did the stair monster. Why would anyone invent a machine to simulate an activity rendered obsolete by the invention of elevators? Tanya told me regular exercise would make me live longer. I can't imagine anything worse.

Day 4

Tanya was waiting for me with her vampire teeth in a full snarl. I can't help it if I was half an hour late—it took me that long just to tie my shoes. She wanted me to lift dumbbells. Not a chance, Tanya.

The world "dumb" must be in there for a reason. I hid in the men's room until she sent Lars looking for me. As punishment she made me try the rowing machine. It sank.

Day 5

I hate Tanya more than any human being has ever hated any other human being in the history of the world. If there was any part of my body not in extreme pain I would hit her with it. She thought it would be a good idea to work on my triceps. Well, I have news for you, Tanya: I don't have triceps. And if you don't want dents in the floor, don't hand me any barbells. I refuse to accept responsibility for the damage. *You* went to sadist school. *You* are to blame. The treadmill flung me back into a science teacher, which hurt like crazy. Why couldn't it have been someone softer, like a music or social studies teacher?

Day 6

Got Tanya's message on my answering machine, wondering where I am. I lacked the strength to use the TV remote, so I watched eleven straight hours of the Weather Channel.

Day 7

Well, that's the week. Thank God that's over. Maybe next time my wife will give me something a little more fun, like free tooth drilling at the dentist's.

For a quick check of exercise intensity levels, review the target zones listed in the following table for people ranging in age from twenty to ninety years. The table presents target zones and maximum heart rates for average, relatively sedentary people. For very fit people, target zones and maximum heart rates would decline very little as they age.

Age	Target Zone (60–80%, beats/minute)	Maximum Heart Rate (100%)
20	120–160	200
25	117–156	195
30	114–152	190
35	111–148	185
40	108–144	180
45	105–140	175
50	102–136	170
55	99–132	165
60	96–128	160
65	93–124	155
70	90–120	150
75	87–116	145
80	84–112	140
85	81–108	135

After six months or more of regular exercising, you can exercise up to 85 percent of your maximum heart rate. However, you do not have to exercise that hard to stay in excellent condition. To check your heart rate during exercise, take your pulse immediately after you stop exercising:

1. As soon as you stop exercising, place the tips of your first two fingers lightly over one of the blood vessels on your neck (carotid arteries) to the left or right of the center of your throat. Another convenient place to determine your heart rate (or pulse) is the inside of your wrist just below the base of your thumb.
2. Count your pulse for ten seconds and multiply by six.
3. If your pulse (heart rate) is below your target zone, consider exercising a little harder next time. If you are above your target zone, exercise a little more easily the next time. If your pulse falls within your target zone, you are doing fine.

Remember, any exercise, even exercise below your target zone, helps promote effective weight control. This recommendation about target zones pertains to maintaining and improving cardiovascular fitness. You may also find it helpful to check your heart rate if your intensity level feels too high. You can check to see if you are in your target zone, and you will probably find that you feel quite uncomfortable when you exercise above your target zone. Decreasing the intensity of your exercising will allow you to exercise for 30 minutes or more.

Duration of Exercise

The American College of Sports Medicine endorses exercise sessions lasting from 30 to 60 minutes. Many people have difficulty maintaining aerobic activities for 30 minutes or more. If you are one of these people, try starting with sessions that last 10 or 15 minutes. Two 15-minute sessions of exercise produce about the same benefits as one 30-minute session. In fact, from a weight-control perspective, you will enjoy better results from frequent exercise for shorter amounts of time than from one long session.

Some confusing theories about the length of exercise sessions have become popular. One concerns "fat burning." It suggests that you won't "burn fat" unless you exercise for long periods of time. This assertion is wrong. When you begin exercising, you begin using calories immediately. The energy consumed by your body initially comes from glucose stored in the muscles. As you exercise for longer periods of time, your body begins dipping into its energy reserves (fat). However, your body must replenish the energy supply it uses. This means that when you consume energy in the form of stored glucose from the muscles, your body will use its stored energy supply to replenish the glucose taken from the muscles. It makes no difference whether you exercise for short bursts of 10 or 15 minutes or for longer periods of 30 to 60 minutes per session. You burn fat in both ways.

Ellen, one of my clients, described how she began exercising for very short periods of time. She then gradually extended the duration of her exercise:

> I began exercising for 15 seconds at a time on my Schwinn Air-Dyne with the oversized seat. I just couldn't seem to stay on that thing for more than a few seconds at a time. Of course, I weighed 340 pounds when I started using it. So I did 15 seconds three times a day. Then I was able to do it longer and longer every day. Now, 190 lost pounds later, I use my Air-Dyne for 30 to 40 minutes every morning. Sometimes I go to an aerobics class or do a fast walk instead. But I do exercise every day, sometimes twice a day. It makes me feel reasonably good. Although I must admit, I would quit it all in a second if I could find some other way of keeping healthy and keeping my weight down. Exercising like I do sure beats the alternative of being so big.

Mode of Exercise

When I was growing up in Brooklyn, New York, in the 1950s, jogging didn't really exist. If you saw a man running down the street, you knew someone else was chasing him. The term "running shoes" also did not exist. The idea of spending as much money for "running shoes" as some people spend on a set of tires still amazes me.

The world has changed a great deal in these last forty years. Options for exercising are everywhere. Health clubs are no longer places for fanatics. They are commonplace in many communities—especially in urban centers. Almost everyone has not only heard of running shoes but owns at least one pair. Joggers run everywhere. Exercising has become part of everyday life.

Which options produce the best outcomes for weight controllers? My clients ask about the benefits of stair-climbing machines versus treadmills. People wonder about exercise equipment they can buy for their homes versus equipment in health clubs. Personal trainers have become another controversial addition to the possibilities for exercising.

Research shows that addressing three elements of exercising seems particularly helpful: convenience, appeal, and social aspects. First, *convenience* affects exercising. If you join a health club twenty miles from your home or twenty miles from work, will you really use it regularly enough? Most people would not. In fact, many health clubs advertise as aggressively as possible to get people to join. The clubs realize that most people will not use the facilities, and their greatest profit comes from people who join and then disappear. Certainly walking, jogging, and in-home exercising are very convenient for most people. When looking at health clubs, consider joining one that requires minimal transportation. If you can find one next door to your job or within walking distance from home, it may be the best buy for you.

Second, the *appeal* of an exercise routine affects your use of it. Do you like walking? Or do you prefer a more social and musical activity, like aerobics classes? Perhaps if you can make a game of your exercising, you will pursue it more effectively. Some people like racquetball and tennis because they enjoy the competition and camaraderie of those sports. You can also make your exercising as enjoyable as possible. Research shows that people who walk or jog exercise more vigorously and consistently if they use a Walkman-type radio and cassette player. Some recent versions include push-button digital tuning that makes switching from station to station very easy. Setting up a treadmill at home is an art form in and of itself. It helps to use earphones (wireless earphones are especially good) connected to the television or to a CD player to provide a variety of distractions. Many people also exercise at home in front of a VCR while watching a rented movie.

More equipment means more money. These are dollars well spent for weight controllers. Many people, however, do not have enough money to spare to buy such high-tech distractions. Various versions of the Walkman-type radio and cassette players, on the other hand, aren't very costly and last a long time.

Finally, *social* aspects of exercise can affect your consistency. If you can walk with a friend or spouse, you may find walking far more enjoyable than solitary journeys. The "loneliness of the long-distance runner" can make it difficult to remain enthusiastic about exercising on your own. In contrast, some people like the time alone that exercise provides. I have heard many people say, "Let me run on that tomorrow morning." These runners use their jogging time to solve problems. Problem solving goes remarkably well when phones aren't ringing and people aren't knocking on the door. If you are one of those people who enjoy the company of others while exercising, social sports such as golf and bowling can add an important dimension to exercising.

My clients tend to prefer treadmills over exercycles. The people who own treadmills seem to use them more frequently. Unfortunately, *Consumer Reports'* engineers found that most lower-cost treadmills do not work very well. They tend to be noisy and break down regularly. You might have to pay $1,000 or so for a high-quality, relatively quiet, and reliable piece of equipment that should last for many years.

Another mode of home exercising involves the use of exercise videotapes. Many of the videotapes on the market, however, contain inappropriate information, and some offer potentially dangerous advice. Two physiologists (experts in exercise) recently evaluated the ten top-selling videotapes. They found that four of the videotapes contained as little as five minutes of aerobic exercise. Two contained none at all! Several of the tapes did not include enough warm-up time. *All* of the tapes that were studied included exercise that the experts strongly advised against. These exercises included "ballistic stretching without adequate warm-up." Ballistic stretching uses sudden, jerky movements, like bouncing. "Static stretching" is vastly preferred because it increases flexibility by slowly stretching a muscle and holding it in that position for several seconds. "Ballistic stretching" can tear or strain muscles very easily. Many of the tapes also included overextension of certain regions of the spine and knee joints. More recent tapes are somewhat better. For example, Kathy Smith has created several safer and more appropriate videotapes (two good ones are *Kathy Smith: Starting Out* and *Kathy Smith's Winning Workout*). In general, you should use exercise videotapes with caution.

Strength Training (Weight Lifting)

It is a little-known fact that by age seventy-four about one-third of all men and two-thirds of all women can't lift a gallon of milk (approximately eight pounds). The average adult loses about six or seven pounds of muscle per decade after that. Most people have one-third fewer muscle cells than they had at age twenty. Also, the muscle cells of seventy-year-olds are smaller than those of a twenty-year-old. Aging, however, does not cause these declines in muscularity. Disuse and sedentary living cause this weakening of the muscles.

In 1990 the American College of Sports Medicine (ACSM) emphasized the importance of resistance training more strongly than ever before. Strength training of moderate intensity (50 to 60 percent of maximal lifting ability) provides important benefits. The ACSM recommends selecting exercises that incorporate many different body parts and different kinds of movements. They suggest performing lifting exercises continuously, using smooth, slow, and controlled motions. Maintaining good posture when lifting weights will help you avoid injury. Only the body part being exercised while lifting the weight should be in motion during a lift. Other body parts should be at rest and stationary when weight lifting. Let's review several other critical questions about weight lifting.

How many repetitions? Eight to twelve repetitions are recommended if you want to improve both strength and endurance. Most exercise experts suggest that if you can lift the weight easily more than twelve times, it is time to add more weight. When you add more weight, go back to eight to twelve repetitions per exercise.

How many sets? The ACSM recommends using 8 to 10 different kinds of weight-lifting exercises per session. If you make only enough time to do one set of each exercise, you will still strengthen your muscles 70 to 80 percent as much as you would by doing multiple sets. A full session of eight or ten exercises, including warm-up time, can take as little as 15 minutes to do.

How many workouts? The ideal strengthening program includes three workouts a week. Squeezing in more than three workouts per week might slow the growth of your muscles. Muscles need a day off to recover from weight training. Interestingly, you can get about 75 percent of the maximum improvement available from weight lifting by working out only twice a week. If you don't have much time, even a single strengthening session per week helps far more than none at all. According to one study, a weekly workout can help you maintain your current levels of strength for several months.

Strength training for the legs? People who do aerobic exercises may not need strengthening exercises for the legs. Most aerobic exercises keep leg muscles in good shape. However, strengthening for the legs may improve your ability to run, play sports, or climb stairs. It can also help older people walk longer distances and may prevent knee and hip injuries.

How much is enough? To keep building strength, you must keep increasing the weights you lift. You can maintain a desired level of strength by simply maintaining twelve repetitions for a particular exercise. If you stop weight lifting, your strength will begin to fade within two weeks. After three to five months, you'll be back to where you started.

What's the procedure for weight lifting? Several guidelines can help you prevent injuries and maximize the benefits of weight lifting. First, it helps if you warm up for a few minutes by doing jumping jacks, jogging in place, and then stretching. Stretch your shoulders, lower back, calves, and the front and back of your thighs. Stretch slowly and steadily to the point of tension, not pain, and hold the position for 3 to 30 seconds.

Second, breathe slowly and steadily during weight lifting. Holding your breath while tensing your muscles can cause light-headedness and even fainting. Exhale as you either lift the weight or raise your body, and inhale as you return to the starting position. Third, perform the repetitions slowly. Each one should take about six seconds—two to lift and four to lower. Jerky movements can cause injury and soreness. Fourth, stop if your muscles hurt. The dictum "No pain, no gain" is both wrong and potentially dangerous. Your muscles should feel fatigued during the last repetitions, but you should not feel sharp or piercing pains in your muscles or joints. If you do feel pain, stop the exercise immediately. Finally, cool down after you exercise by doing a few minutes of walking or light jogging, followed by stretching again.

It is helpful to have a well-qualified personal trainer show you proper techniques and a range of weight-lifting exercises to consider. A personal trainer should have a master's degree in physical education or exercise physiology and certification by the American Council on Exercise.

Exercise versus Daily Activity: Everything Counts
Everyday activities, aside from exercising, also consume calories. The following are some common activities and the calories expended per minute by a 150-pound person:

Activity	Calories Burned per Minute
Car washing	4.0
Gardening	5.0
Grocery shopping	4.0
Mowing lawn (pushing power mower)	5.0
Painting house	5.0
Raking leaves	4.0

Activity	Calories Burned per Minute
Shoveling snow	8.0
Sweeping	4.0
Vacuuming	3.3

You can see that many of our daily activities expend significant numbers of calories. These numbers suggest the dictum Move whenever and wherever possible. *If you want to lose weight and maintain weight loss, find creative ways of staying active.* One of my clients did this by buying a desk that she could use only while standing up. She knew that standing burned twice as many calories as sitting and used this knowledge to her advantage. Another client who worked in a school decided to avoid the elevator. She took the long way down corridors to talk to colleagues and students. People who work in stores can avoid escalators and use stairs whenever the alternative presents itself. Parking farther rather than closer to your destination provides additional opportunities for walking.

These everyday methods of expending calories really add up. Studies of overweight children in camp showed that they expended fewer calories playing the same games and sports as children who were not overweight. This indicates that people with weight problems may tend to avoid expending energy in everyday activities more than those who do not have weight problems. Some recent studies of people in major cities also support this. When given the opportunity to take the stairs or an escalator or elevator, overweight people take the stairs less frequently than people who are not overweight. Every time you take a more active, rather than a sedentary, alternative pathway, you burn calories and elevate your metabolic rate. Everything counts.

Excuses, Excuses

I met one of my childhood friends for dinner last year. I had not seen Tom for twenty years. Tom looked good and was happy with his family life and his work as a pharmacist. We talked about various things, including exercise. Tom noticed that I had lost a considerable amount of weight and seemed to be in excellent physical condition compared to the way he remembered me. He asked the usual questions about "my secret."

I discussed the importance of exercise in my life. As a health professional, he was fully aware of the value of exercising. However, he told me, "I really wish I had time for exercise." I talked about the idea of making time for exercise rather than thinking of it as an option. He argued that he "just didn't have time for it."

When I probed about this time constraint, Tom indicated that he believed exercise would interfere with his ability to earn a decent living. He wanted to work more and more hours every year to keep increasing his income. It turns out that he and his wife made a more than satisfactory income and had no major financial pressures. In fact, his wife is a successful physician, and they earn more money than 99 percent of the households in the United States. I asked, "Wouldn't you and your family be better off if you were healthier and happier than if you made an extra few thousand dollars per year by working additional hours that you could use for exercising?" Tom argued that he and his wife do not like to take out loans when they buy something like a car. I replied incredulously, "You mean that you feel a 'need' to pay for your cars in cash and that's the reason you don't exercise?" "I guess so," responded Tom weakly.

Exercise takes time and requires some sacrifice. Tom decided that the "sacrifice" of taking out a loan to buy a new car every ten years (which he and his family could easily afford) outweighed the benefits of exercising. This is a remarkable piece of rationalization.

Like most struggling weight controllers, you've probably found some creative ways to talk yourself out of exercising. What are your top ten reasons for *not* exercising? How have you argued yourself back into brisk walks in the morning or some other form regular activity? In twenty-five years of helping people debate themselves successfully on this point, I've discovered a few of the better arguments and counterarguments. You may find reviewing some of these helpful when trying to convince yourself to take this important step toward controlling your weight more effectively:

I'm too tired.	Exercising will energize me. I am unwilling to give in to a temporary feeling of tiredness.
I need more sleep.	It would be nice to get more sleep. Exercising will help me sleep better. I can go to sleep earlier or sleep longer tomorrow. Being a little sleepy won't hurt me.
I have more important things to do.	Making time for myself is as important as anything else. I can work more efficiently if I exercise and stay healthy. I can even think about my work while exercising to jump-start it when I get back.
I'm too busy.	What's more important to me? Exercise deserves to be a high priority in my life. It does take time. It takes time to invest in myself, my health, my well-being, my future.
I'd rather relax.	Just because I'd rather relax doesn't mean that's the best thing for me to do now. It's more important to fulfill my commitment to losing weight.

I don't feel good enough.	Unless I have a fever or I am deathly ill, I know it's safe for me to exercise.
	I can always exercise at a lower intensity than usual. I can walk instead of run, or I can jog slowly instead of at my usual pace. I can do at least 15 or 20 minutes of something.
	I'd rather reduce my exercise than do none at all.
I'm just not motivated to do it.	I do not have to wait for some magical level of "motivation." I can "just do it!" If I think about why I want to exercise, that will increase my motivation.
I'll do it later (or tomorrow).	If I convince myself to do it later, I might not do it at all. If I get it out of the way, I'll feel better.
It's not a big deal if I miss one day.	Every day counts. If I don't make today count, what makes me think I will make tomorrow count? My commitment is a commitment to every day. Every day counts.

Preventing and Managing Injuries

Have injuries ever interfered with your exercise habits? When people injure an ankle or a back, it can take a long time, if not forever, for them to get back to regular exercising. Even minor and common illnesses, including colds, can change the momentum of consistent exercising. Exercising takes time, costs money, and interferes with your life to a significant degree. When we become sick or injured, living without exercising becomes normal. This increases the challenge of working exercise back into a complicated life. This makes sense: There is nothing crazy or neurotic about not exercising. It takes devotion, commitment, and focusing to make exercising a part of your life.

You have choices about managing illnesses and injuries. First, you can either expect some injuries and illnesses to interfere with your exercising or you can just hope "It won't happen to me." The latter choice almost never works well. You can plan more effectively when your expectations fit reality better. What will you do *if* you get sick? How would you manage a back or knee injury? It helps to plan for these common problems.

Second, you can take an aggressive approach to managing illnesses and injuries or a more conservative approach. The aggressive approach usually includes exercising sooner than you think you can. Doctors I've consulted often recommend resting when fevers go to 100 degrees or more. When fevers get below 100 degrees and you feel capable of some easy exercise, like walking, you can go for it. "Exercise a day or two before you think you can," I have heard from some very knowledgeable physicians. Consider your reaction to a doctor suggesting the more conservative (and typical) "Rest until you're feeling much better." Do you simply follow that advice? You could. You could also challenge it gently by asking if you could go for a several-mile walk or do some other low-impact workout sooner, rather than later.

Consider asking your doctor specifically about the medical risks of exercising at various levels of intensity and various durations. "Can I walk three miles? Five miles? Slowly jog three miles? Use a step machine for 20 minutes? Play doubles tennis?" "Yes" or "no" answers are not good enough. Try to find out the advantages and risks of various alternatives, then decide what to do. It's your body, and your commitment to weight control. If you manage it as actively as you can, you'll probably feel better about it.

You can consult your doctor about illness and exercise, but who do you consult for some of the more common exercise-related maladies? Problems with knees, backs, hips, and feet plague middle-aged exercisers as well as many highly trained twenty-year-old athletes. All athletic teams at the college level use athletic trainers to help mend these maladies quickly and avoid unnecessary damage. At Olympic events, dozens of athletic trainers help the athletes stay competitive despite various strains and sprains. You can get similar assistance at physical therapy centers. Almost all hospitals have such centers. Sometimes these centers are located in hospital rehabilitation or orthopedic clinics.

Some large-scale studies also support the effectiveness of chiropractors specifically for back problems. Sometimes foot problems lead to knee problems and/or to hip and back problems. Podiatrists can help when feet become uncooperative.

Consider investigating physical therapy, chiropractic, and podiatric alternatives. Each approach has advantages and disadvantages, depending on the nature of the problem. The key to feeling better is—you guessed it—persistence. Try to pursue various alternatives until some approach makes sense and really helps. It is frustrating. The healing arts remain more art than science, unfortunately. Support from others sometimes helps, but even without support, remember the critical role exercise plays in effective weight control. You can find lower-impact (or less intense) alternatives when injuries occur (walking or swimming instead of jogging or playing tennis, for example). You can refuse to stop moving whenever possible. You can manage your weight with an imperfect body. You cannot manage your weight by becoming or staying sedentary.

Safety Tips

Perhaps the best way of managing injuries is to avoid them. The American Heart Association suggests the following helpful hints:

- Stretch, warm up, and cool down.
- Build up your level of activity gradually
- Listen to your body for early warning signs.
- Be aware of possible signs of heart problems.
- Take appropriate precautions for special weather conditions.

Stretch, warm up, and cool down. Warming up for several minutes gives your body a chance to get ready for more vigorous exercise. Start at a slow to medium pace and gradually increase it for several minutes. Warm-ups can include jogging in place or just moving around slowly and beginning to orient your body to exercise.

Stretching exercises are a very important part of the warm-up. Do stretching exercises slowly and in a steady, rhythmical way. Many different stretches are possible. Here are four that are widely used:

- *Wall push.* Stand one to two feet away from a wall. Lean forward, pushing against the wall, keeping your heels flat. Count to ten, then rest. Repeat one or two times.
- *Palm touch.* Stand with your knees slightly bent. Bend from the waist and try to touch your palms either to your ankles or to the floor. Do not bounce. Count to ten, then rest. Repeat this one or two times. If you have lower back problems, do this exercise with your legs crossed.
- *Toe touch.* Place your right leg on a stair, chair, or other object. Keeping your other leg straight, lean forward slowly to touch your right toe with your right hand ten times. Then do this with your left hand ten times. Again, do not bounce. Switch legs and repeat with each hand. Repeat the entire exercise one or two times.
- *Shoulder blade scratch.* Reach back with one arm as if to scratch your shoulder blade. Use the other hand to extend the stretch. Alternate arms. Repeat one or two times.

Cool down for several minutes after exercising. The cooldown should progress slowly and gradually. For example, swim more slowly or change to a more leisurely stroke. You can also cool down by walking for several minutes after a jog. Cooling down allows your body to relax gradually. It also helps remove buildups of the by-products of exercising that accumulate in the muscles. Abrupt stopping can cause dizziness and cramping or muscle soreness later in the day. Consider repeating your stretching and warm-up exercises to loosen up your muscles after an exercise session.

Build up your level of activity gradually. Starting out slowly helps you avoid overexertion. This decreases the likelihood of injury. Remember, even if you walk at a slow pace, you accomplish much more than staying sedentary.

Listen to your body for early warning signs. You can feel pains in your joints, feet, ankles, and legs quite easily when you're just getting used to exercising. Minor muscle and joint injuries can be treated readily by aspirin and rest. When you feel pain, discontinue what you are doing. If you feel a pain in your ankle when running, for example, try slowing down for a while and seeing if the pain goes away. If it persists, stop running. Some discomforts are perfectly normal during exercising. It may take a while for you to recognize the difference between normal discomforts and potentially problematic pains.

Be aware of possible signs of heart problems. Pain or pressure in the left or midchest area, left neck, shoulder, or arm during or just after exercising can be a sign of a heart problem. These sorts of pains can also occur due to the normal strains of exercising. For example, a "stitch" is a common, relatively sharp pain that occurs below the bottom of your ribs. It is a cramping of some muscles due to a temporary lack of oxygen to those muscles. Stitches stop when you slow down. Heart problems do not cause stitches. On the other hand, sudden dizziness, cold sweats, and fainting are signs of much more dangerous problems. If any of these things happen during or immediately after exercising, get medical attention right away.

Take appropriate precautions for special weather conditions.
When it is hot and humid outside, consider exercising less intensely
than normal for a week or so until you adapt to the heat. It also helps
to exercise during the cooler parts of the day, such as early morning
or early evening after the sun has gone down. Fluid intake becomes
especially important under conditions in which you might become
dehydrated (for example, when traveling or during particularly hot
days). On such hot days, you might think you also need extra salt.
Actually, you do not need extra salt; you get enough salt in your diet.
Also, if you maintain a good level of physical fitness, your body learns
to conserve salt, and your sweat consists mostly of water.

On very hot and sunny days, the possibility of heat stroke is a concern. Signs of heat stroke include feeling dizzy, weak, light-headed,
and excessively tired. Also watch for a sudden decrease in sweating
and a rapid increase in body temperature. If you feel sensations very
much like these, get yourself to a cooler place as soon as possible,
drink some fluids, rest, and seek medical attention.

Dress appropriately for hot weather. It helps to wear very light,
loose-fitting clothing. Rubberized or plastic suits, sweatshirts, and
sweatpants do nothing but increase your risk of heat stroke. Such
clothing does not help you lose weight any faster. It does make you
sweat more, but the weight you lose in fluids by sweating is quickly
replaced as soon as you begin drinking fluids again.

On cold days, wear one less layer of clothing than you would if
you were outside but not exercising. Some people find that they can
wear a couple of layers less than they normally would. Several layers
of clothing work better than a single layer of heavier clothes. You
can wear old mittens, gloves, or cotton socks to protect your hands.
Some of my clients wear inexpensive cotton garden gloves while
walking or running. Since up to 40 percent of your body's heat is lost
through your neck and head, wearing a comfortable hat seems especially advisable in cold weather.

Remember that rainy, icy, and snowy days make for special hazards
for exercisers. Persistent weight controllers develop a variety of alter-

native means of exercising that allow for these weather conditions. They may use indoor tracks or machines at health clubs, play racquetball, take tennis lessons, or use their own treadmills or exercycles.

Other miscellaneous tips. Here are a few additional hints for safe exercising:

- Avoid strenuous exercise for at least two hours after eating a meal. It also aids digestion to wait about twenty minutes before eating following an exercise session.
- Proper equipment can prevent a variety of injuries. This includes good running shoes for walkers or runners and goggles to protect eyes for racquetball, handball, and squash players.
- Hard and uneven surfaces, such as cement or rough fields, cause more injuries than smoother surfaces. Soft, even surfaces such as level grass fields, dirt paths, and tracks for running are better for your feet and joints.
- When you walk, run, or jog, try to land on your heels rather than on the balls of your feet. This minimizes the strain on your feet, knees, and lower legs. Try to keep your feet as close to the ground as possible without tripping. This method helps you land on your heels more so than on your toes.
- Walkers and joggers get hit by bicycles and cars more often than you might think. It helps to wear brightly colored clothes and reflecting bands on your clothes and shoes. Drivers will notice you more if you face them. That also allows you to protect yourself more directly. The basic message is: Exercise defensively. Bicyclists can prevent injuries by wearing a helmet, using a light, and putting reflectors on their wheels for night riding. It also helps to ride in the direction of traffic and to avoid busy streets.

One definition of middle age is: fifteen years older than you are now. Forty years old represents another threshold for middle age that researchers use. Many people concerned about weight have

crossed the magic forty-year-old threshold. Middle-aged weight controllers commonly experience minor injuries. Ankles get sprained,
backs get painful, hips start hurting, and knees swell up. Every ath-
lete experiences these problems as well. Remember that weight controllers are very much like athletes in training. You are attempting to
push your body to a place it doesn't want to go. Your brain can take
over and nudge your body forward, despite the inevitable aches and
pains along the way.

One of my clients, who prefers to remain anonymous, struggled
mightily with developing a consistent exercise plan. She created the
following poem during the height of her struggle.

With Wont's, You Can't

If you can't run every morning,
    then run in the evening.
If you can't run,
    then walk briskly.
If you can't walk briskly,
    just walk slowly or treadmill or bike or swim.
If you can't do any of this, let's face it,
    you "can't" because you "won't."
You "can't" walk,
    because you won't make it a priority.
You can succeed with some can'ts,
    but not with won'ts.
Won't you make yours better every day?

SIX

❖

Managing Stress

**Truth #8: You can manage stress
without overeating or underexercising.**

Take a minute to think about the successful achievements of your
life. What was your life like when you were most successful in school
or at work or in some creative project?

You probably managed various challenges effectively while you
were succeeding. Family and friends may have supported you. You
somehow handled the emotional demands of everyday life with
calmness and efficiency. Performing well on the job, in school, in
sports, and in weight control all require this kind of effective stress
management.

This chapter will help you understand how to handle your life in
an orderly and calm state, thereby allowing you to succeed at weight
control. You will learn how to define stress and stressors and how to
improve your coping skills.

Stress and Stressors

One way to bring the issues of stress management to life is to consider some examples of people who managed stress effectively and

those who did not. The experiences of Sylvia and Sue provide a sharp contrast regarding stress management.

Sylvia's Stress

Sylvia began her weight-loss effort in earnest three years ago, when she was twenty-nine. She was a strikingly attractive woman who was successful at her busy career in journalism. Yet she was approximately 20 pounds overweight, and her standards of attractiveness made this 20 pounds almost intolerable. She noted, for example, "I just can't stand myself like this! I feel gross and annoyed at myself every single day, practically every single minute. It seems I do nothing but think about food and feeling fat. I've got to get beyond this craziness."

Sylvia lived by herself and, therefore, had good control of her home environment. Her very active social life, though, kept her out of her home and placed her in bars and restaurants quite often. On many occasions, she stayed out late and drank enough wine or beer to produce a mild hangover in the morning. As a relatively junior journalist in a big city like Chicago, Sylvia was called to work on stories that sometimes took her far past her normal working hours and got her on the road, traveling widely. Her hours fluctuated tremendously depending upon the kind of stories she was following.

Sylvia's condo reflected the chaos she experienced through much of her life. It was cluttered with unopened mail and piles of magazines, and her closets looked as if small tornadoes had landed in them repeatedly. She was also under serious financial pressure, having spent more money than she earned on such things as clothes, partying, and the condo itself. At the end of every month, Sylvia found herself juggling checks coming in and checks going out with considerable distress.

Sylvia began her work with me by keeping careful track of her eating and exercising. However, she found it very difficult to exercise, even to take half-hour brisk walks, on those days when she woke up with a hangover and was scurrying about trying to get to work on time. Also, she "didn't have time" to look up fat grams, get very specific about her eating, or keep written records. After one week of reasonable progress and a two-pound weight loss, Sylvia began noticing that her weight didn't move downward. Her self-monitoring grew sketchy, and she started to miss some appointments with me. Over the subsequent year, she showed up sporadically, always feeling desperate to begin a renewed effort to improve her weight control. By the end of the year her weight was approximately the same as it was at the beginning of the year. She discontinued her sessions with me, but she came back every once in a while over the following two years. Her drinking and lifestyle remained in relatively poor control, as did her weight.

Compare Sylvia's story to Sue's. Can you see some similarities to yourself in either case? If you swirl like Sylvia, this chapter could help you develop some of the serenity that characterizes Sue.

Sue's Stress Management

Sue was thirty-one when she began her treatment program with me, three years ago. She had been married for several years, had no children, and had made a very serious commitment to lose 30 pounds. She was very well organized in all aspects of her life. Her finances were stable and she was generally happy and content. Her husband supported her efforts to lose weight by exercizing with her and cheering her on as she learned a new lifestyle.

Sue bought a treadmill and set it up in a convenient location, facing a VCR, and purchased wireless headphones. She meticulously kept written records of all aspects of her eating and exercising. She found it useful to look up and record total calories and fat grams consumed. She and her husband both liked to cook, and they went through recipes they found on the Internet that promoted low-fat or no-fat eating.

Sue's condo looked orderly and comfortable. She had no difficulties attending her sessions on time, every time. She also reported that at least part of her enjoyed the discipline that weight control demands.

Sue lost approximately 25 of the 30 pounds she had intended to lose. She made this progress within a year and has continued to return for sessions every two to four weeks to "keep the focus." Her weight has remained stable over these last two years, despite occasional demands from her job to travel and various challenges from vacations.

Definitions

Sylvia experienced a variety of complex emotional responses to the demands of her life. These complex negative responses are defined as "stress." The term "stressor" describes the cause of those responses. In Sylvia's case, the causes of the stress (the stressors) include her demanding job with its long and variable hours, as well as her chaotic and disorganized style of managing her life. Stress encompasses negative feelings such as frustration, tension, irritability, hostility, and anger. These feelings emerge as reactions to specific stressors, such as unusual demands from work or travel or family.

Degrees of Stress

Take a look at the types of stress described below. How many of those responses have you experienced that were directly related to a specific environmental demand in the last few weeks? If you recognize many of those responses and can tie them to specific demands, you are experiencing a high level of stress. These unhappy and frustrated feelings can make the "aggressive self-protectiveness" needed for successful weight control difficult to obtain. How can you make time in your life for exercise, keep your food choices in control, and stay focused and optimistic about weight control in the face of these unhappy feelings and reactions? Perhaps it would help to have a better understanding of the types of situations that create these challenging and frustrating reactions.

Stress Responses

Physical

- Appetite change
- Decreased attention span
- Fatigue
- Sleep problems
- Headaches
- Weight change
- Colds
- Stomach upsets
- Muscle aches
- Heart pounding
- Physical accidents
- Teeth grinding
- Restlessness
- Skin problems
- Foot tapping
- Finger drumming
- Increased drug, alcohol, tobacco use

Emotional

- Anxiety
- Frustration
- Anger
- Mood swings
- Temper tantrums
- Nightmares
- Crying spells
- Irritability
- Blues
- Depression
- Worrying
- Discouragement
- Unhappiness
- Emptiness
- Cynicism
- Apathy

Mental

- Unproductiveness
- Forgetfulness
- Boredom
- Dullness of senses
- Confusion

Interpersonal

- Distrustful
- Isolation
- Intolerance
- Resentful
- Lonely

Mental

- Poor concentration
- Spacing out
- Feeling like nothing matters
- Silly mistakes
- Ineffectiveness

Interpersonal

- Overly critical
- Clamming up
- Decreased sex drive
- Nagging
- Decreased intimacy
- Using people
- Cynical
- Unforgiving
- Decreased contacts with friends

Types of Stressors

All stressors seem unpredictable and/or uncontrollable. Sylvia gets involved in a story and suddenly it becomes something she has to work on well into the evening hours. Or she gets to the end of a month and suddenly realizes she does not have enough money to pay her bills. When you lose your keys or forget a phone number that you wanted to call immediately, you can start feeling the frustration and annoyance that characterize stress. These events occur without warning and are nearly impossible to control.

Think for a moment about events that have caused you stress recently. You may notice that some of them seem more uncontrollable than unpredictable, or vice versa. For example, your dog barks whenever a cat strolls by. You cannot predict when a cat will appear, but you can control your dog's barking once it starts. On the other hand, the fact that rush-hour traffic produces annoyances is very predictable, but it is impossible for you to control. Because many events are unpredictable or uncontrollable or both, it would take hundreds of pages to discuss them all. Instead, let's consider how major "life events" and minor "daily hassles" affect you.

Major life events. Major life events that disrupt routines and decrease feelings of security produce the most stress. For example, most people function very poorly in many ways if a family member dies, if a spouse leaves them, or if they are fired from a job.

The impact of these negative life events depends directly on your specific reactions to them. Think about how your friends have reacted when an important relationship of theirs broke up. One friend may rehash what went wrong and feel severely rejected and depressed. Another friend in the same situation may recover quickly and try to find another partner. In a similar vein, some people get very involved when the United States participates in a military action. They become absorbed with the event, watch the news late into the evening, and find it extremely distressing. Other people take such national emergencies much more lightly. Your view of the importance of events in your life and the world can determine if these major life events will produce stress for you.

Daily hassles. Daily annoyances or hassles can produce as much stress as some major life events. Consider the degree to which the following hassles affected your stress levels in recent weeks:

- Being interrupted while talking
- Experiencing problems with children
- Being ignored by others
- Having someone break a promise or appointment
- Having a minor argument with spouse, friend, coworker
- Being embarrassed
- Performing poorly at a task
- Doing something you are unskilled at
- Being unable to complete a task
- Being late
- Failing to understand something
- Having someone fail to knock at your door
- Worrying about someone else's problems

- Being interrupted during a task
- Being crowded or pushed
- Having a minor accident (broke something, tore clothing)
- Experiencing bad weather
- Having difficulty in traffic
- Being criticized
- Becoming fearful
- Misplacing something
- Forgetting something
- Doing something that you did not want to do

You may have felt some discomfort just reading and remembering when these events happened to you. When two or more of these events occur in one day, most people react quite negatively. Do you think it would affect your food choices if you felt that you were late all day for your appointments or you were constantly interrupted in the tasks you focused upon during that day? Wouldn't you be a bit more likely to make less thoughtful choices about food and more likely to eat "comfort food"?

Clearly, both minor daily hassles and major life events produce challenges to your weight-control efforts. If you can find a way of quickly mastering the impact of these stressors, you will become a more effective weight controller.

Techniques for Managing Stress
How would you react to the following situation: You had to work very late last night and could only get about half of your normal amount of sleep. Would you: (a) Skip your usual morning workout and just grab whatever was available for breakfast or (b) get up early enough to work out anyway (perhaps doing a shorter than usual workout) and then have your usual breakfast?

Tiredness often increases problems with eating and decreases exercising. Some people, however, can manage this kind of stressor and many others without skipping a beat on their weight-control program. Most people cannot do that. Let's consider several characteristics of people who handle stress very effectively, the role that help from others can play, and a technique called "stress inoculation" that can prepare you to handle stressors more effectively.

Hardiness

Explorers, pioneers, and lumberjacks seem hardy. But can you imagine a hardy lawyer or a hardy business executive? Psychologist Suzanne Kobasa and her colleagues found quite a few hardy lawyers and business executives. These hardy professionals often did not look like gruff pioneers, but they responded to stressors very effectively. Hardy people survive and flourish under stress.

Three Cs define hardiness: *commitment, control,* and *challenge.* To explain these three Cs, let us consider the case of a male executive who just learned that he had to transfer to a new job in a completely new city. The executive, Mr. Mobile, must now face the challenge of working with new people, finding a new home, helping his family adjust to a new neighborhood and new schools, learning new job skills, and getting around in a new city. Because Mr. Mobile is *committed,* he approaches this difficult life event with a sense of purpose. He does not passively allow the newness of his surroundings to overwhelm him. Instead, he actively explores the new job and the new city. He and Ms. Mobile, his wife, spend several hours reading a city map and driving around town to become more familiar with the city. Mr. Mobile even takes the same approach to his new office building. He walks around the building, trying to meet as many new people as possible. Mr. Mobile also sees the new job as another chance for self-improvement. He uses it to learn new skills and to become a better executive. In other words, he finds meaning in the challenge of the new position.

Mr. Mobile sees himself as *controlling* his life. Although the new job places him in a strange new world, he tries to influence what goes on there. He works hard and accomplishes a lot. Mr. Mobile does not believe that he controls everything about this new job, but he does know that hard work, listening to other people, and being open to new learning pays off. Mr. Mobile recognizes that he can control at least some important aspects of his environment, regardless of the stressors he encounters.

Mr. Mobile also enjoys the *challenge* of the job transfer. He recognizes that change is normal in life. He views changes as opportunities that challenge him to grow. Some people fear change because they are afraid that they may not function well in new circumstances. They would rather adjust to stressors than try to become more competent. Mr. Mobile, on the other hand, seeks competence. Merely "adjusting" bores him.

Kobasa found that people like Mr. Mobile, who are committed to their lives and work, who believe they can control their fates, and who see stressors as positive challenges, manage stress very effectively. "Hardy" lawyers and executives remain much healthier than their less hardy colleagues, even when faced with many stressors.

Carin, one of my weight-control clients, demonstrated a less hardy approach to a major conflict at work. Carin had been exercising effectively and eating approximately 1,200 calories and 20 fat grams. When the conflict emerged and became especially severe, she found herself eating a lunch consisting of garlic bread, pasta with heavy cheese sauce, and high-fat ice cream. Carin recognized her response to the stressor from work. She continued her self-monitoring, including writing down both calories and fat grams from her problematic lunch. She and I discussed a method of handling the problem at work, about which she then became energized. Carin had felt unable to control the conflict at work and felt victimized by it. After she and I talked, she had an alternative plan that could begin resolving the problem. She felt much better after developing this plan and, for the first time in a week, went for an exercise walk and began sleeping restfully again. The work problem was eventually resolved, as most of these rather severe stressors usually are after a while. Carin felt a lot better because she accepted the challenge posed by her problem and took control of it.

Can you become a hardier person? How can you take charge of your life? How can you attack problems rather than retreat from them? Try responding to stressors by asking yourself a few questions that direct you to take charge of the situation. For example, you can ask:

- What can I do to eliminate this stressor?
- How can I look at this problem as an opportunity for growth?
- In what way does this stressor tell me something about my goals in life?
- How can I use this situation to improve my competence?

Becoming hardier also involves a little help from your friends. Mr. Mobile was not alone when he made the switch from his old job to his new one. His family cared about him and helped him make the change more smoothly. As discussed in the next section, family and friends can help a great deal—especially in the face of stressors.

A Little Help from Your Friends

People who have good relationships with others suffer fewer medical and emotional problems than more isolated people. People who get good support from others even live longer than those without good connections to other people. A study of seven thousand adults in Alameda County, California, for example, showed that people who lacked relationships with others died at a younger age than those who were married, had frequent contacts with friends and neighbors, and belonged to social clubs or religious groups.

Support from others can reduce the effects of various stressors:

- Women who had another person with them during labor and childbirth experienced fewer complications than did women who did not have a husband, relative, or friend present. The women in the supported group gave birth sooner, were more likely to be awake after delivery, and played with their babies for longer amounts of time than the unsupported group.

• Social support helped men who lost their jobs. Men with good support reported fewer illnesses and less depression than men who did not have adequate support from others following the loss of their jobs.

• Support by parents and hospital staff helped children adjust more effectively to surgery.

• Recovery from heart attacks was improved when people had spouses, friends, and relatives around them.

How do your family and friends support you? How do they help? What do they give you or do for you? The way most people answer these questions indicates that they need more than just the presence of other people; they need people around who actively show that they care.

People show their support in three ways. Family and friends provide us with emotional comforting, helpful information, and material goods such as money or food. All three of these qualities of support can help you manage stress effectively.

Emotional support. People provide emotional support when they:

• listen and talk things over when you want to feel that someone understands you;

• allow you to talk freely about your problems and private thoughts;

• show confidence in you and encourage you.

Informational support. People provide you with informational support when they:

- give you advice you can count on;
- give you names of people who can do very competent work (good doctors and lawyers, for example);
- give you good ideas about personal and family problems.

Material support. People provide you with material support when they:

- look after your belongings (like plants or pets) if you have to leave town for a few days;
- help you get to a doctor if you can't get yourself to one;
- lend you money when you really need it.

Part of stress management includes knowing when and whom to ask for help. Can you identify who you can and do use for support among your family members, neighbors, and coworkers? Does your support network include especially good listeners and very reliable people? When life's little stressors increase, leaning on others helps. Friends and family can provide information, material goods, and emotional support. Their job of helping often becomes easier when we ask for the specific kind of help we want.

Sometimes when you ask for help, you don't get it. Social support doesn't always happen just because you have a spouse who "should" be in the business of providing such support. Consider the case of Judy's battles with Bob, below.

Judy's Battles with Bob—and Then Food

Judy and Bob had been married for four tumultuous years. Judy was a successful journalist for a major newspaper and Bob was an accountant at a large firm in the same city. They both had busy professional lives filled with demands and challenges. They often devoted more time to their professions than to their relationship. They seemed to fight about almost everything, and food was no exception.

Judy decided to work conscientiously to improve her eating and exercising habits. She was approximately 40 pounds overweight when she began this quest. Bob was also somewhat overweight, but he did not want to make it a priority in his life. When Judy began eating lower-fat foods and making more and more time for exercising, Bob objected. They began fighting about what to eat and, more specifically, about what Judy should eat. After several weeks of these skirmishes, Judy laid down the law to Bob: "I am going to decide what I eat and you have to live with it. If I want your ideas about it, I'll ask. This is important to me and I want you to let me make these changes." Bob conceded Judy's right to manage her own body. The skirmishes decreased and a peaceful, although somewhat uneasy, state emerged.

Over the course of the next year, Judy lost almost all of the 40 pounds and became a committed exerciser. She used her health club membership very effectively. She found that exercising provided a good outlet for her stressful life. Judy often talked to Bob about this and encouraged him to consider using this facility to help himself as well. Bob resisted and never accompanied Judy to the club.

One day Judy discovered that Bob had had an affair with a woman at his office. Judy's relationship with Bob had never been great, but it had become a convenient alternative to loneliness. All of that changed very quickly. Judy saw Bob's violation of their commitment to each other as a major and crushing disappointment. She and Bob argued and fought with an intensity she'd never known she had within her. During this time, food and exercising became "unimportant" to Judy. "Nothing else mattered," she told me. "I just didn't care." She ate whatever happened to be available and she "just didn't feel like" exercising anymore. It didn't take long for the weight to come back on and for the old habits to re-emerge in full force.

Perhaps your conflicts in key relationships are less dramatic than Judy and Bob's. Yet even minor disagreements can produce critical lapses. In addition, many spouses try to meddle too much in the life of the weight controller. They may see the weight controller eating high-fat foods or may notice the weight controller decreasing his or her exercising for a few days. When family members use these observations to pressure the weight controller to get back on track, this usually backfires. "I'll show you!" can become a terrific motivator for eating cookies and ice cream.

Because many families have problems with meddling, interfering, or trying to "help too much," I developed the following guidelines for spouses and family members. You may find it useful to photocopy this list and give it to your spouse or family members. This information gently shows significant others *how to help without interfering*.

How to Support a Weight Controller's Efforts

Losing weight and keeping it off is a very difficult process. You can make it easier for your spouse, friend, or partner. Here are several suggestions that will help you support and encourage the weight controllers in your life.

General Attitude

- *Be positive.* Convey to the weight controller that even though it is very difficult to control weight, you believe he or she can do it. This attitude will boost the person's self-confidence while acknowledging the difficulties. Avoid negative comments, criticism, and coercion. These are unhelpful and demoralizing and will create negative feelings between you and the weight controller. This, in turn, could cause him or her to eat more—not less—and thwart the likelihood of success in the long run.
- *Be reinforcing.* Acknowledge the weight controller's accomplish-

ments. Compliments, attention, encouragement, and tangible reinforcement (like little gifts) can help him or her stay motivated and adhere to the plan. Remember, be sincere; superficiality will be interpreted as condescending and aversive.

- *Be realistic.* Weight control requires tremendous effort and skill to overcome strong biological forces. People who are trying to lose weight must adopt eating and exercise patterns that are much more stringent than normal. Don't expect the weight controller to be perfect, or even close to perfect. Occasional slips of overeating, inactivity, weight gain, and failure to adhere to plans will occur. Help the weight controller learn from these experiences rather than dwell on them as "failures."

- *Communicate.* Occasionally inquire about the weight controller's progress. Ask him or her how you can help, thereby complimenting the weight controller's individual efforts. Be open to discussing the challenges of weight control and to assisting in solving problems.

Managing Food

- Increase the amount of nutritious, low-fat foods available to the weight controller.

- Do *not* encourage the weight controller to eat foods that he or she is trying to avoid (for example, refrain from saying, "Let's go out for ice cream," or "Oh, come on, a little bit isn't going to hurt you").

- Help the weight controller prepare foods and recipes in a low-fat way. Encourage experimentation and adventure.

- Adopt appropriate eating habits such as not eating when full, eating appropriate portions, eating in a slow and deliberate fashion, eating regularly or on a schedule, limiting snacking, and limiting the number of eating situations. You may not have a weight problem, but better eating habits may improve your health and will support the weight controller's efforts.

- Plan activities with the weight controller that do not revolve around food (for example, sporting events, concerts, games).
- When you go to a restaurant with the weight controller, select places that make low-fat and low-sugar eating as pleasant as possible.

Promoting Exercise

- Plan activities with the weight controller that involve exercise (for example, walking, hiking, sports).
- Become an exercise partner. You will reap the same physical benefits as your partner.
- Support and encourage the weight controller's individual efforts to exercise.

You can't expect your significant others to provide the kind of support suggested in these guidelines without lapsing, occasionally, back into their former patterns. When this occurs, as it inevitably does, you will do yourself the most good by handling it in a gentle and understanding manner. For example, if your spouse becomes a bit negative or criticizes a food choice that you made, try to avoid an angry outburst. Instead, say something like, "I don't think it helps me when you are negative like that. Remember, no one does weight control perfectly."

Your sources of support also require some maintenance from you. It is very important to give as well as receive support. To do this, you may wish to look for signs from others that they feel stressed. Try to notice when your friends and key family members reach out in your direction. They may start calling you more often or asking you to spend time with them. You may even feel annoyed about having to manage their requests for your time and attention. When feeling such annoyance, think of your efforts as depositing money in a savings account. You may wish to provide support for your significant others even when such efforts add stress to your life.

That nurturing can pay off with a huge dividend when you find yourself wanting help.

Stress Inoculation

Psychologist Don Meichenbaum has developed a useful approach to handling major stressors. This technique, called stress inoculation, builds "psychological antibodies." Stress inoculation has helped people control anger, improve test taking, improve social skills, decrease anxiety about public speaking, decrease anxiety associated with performing music, and decrease fear of flying. It can help you improve your weight control. The procedure includes an educational phase and a coping self-talk phase.

Education about the stressor. In this phase, important information about the stressor is provided. For example, children going to their first dental appointment may not know what will happen there. A friend may have told them that it hurts or that a big person in a white coat will yank out their teeth with a pair of pliers. Just learning what happens in a real dental visit often helps young patients adapt to that difficult situation. In a similar way, many people lack information about a variety of stressors. Students often do not know the best strategies for taking tests; medical patients often have serious misconceptions about their illnesses or about hospitals and treatments; and, more generally, people often do not ask enough questions to learn about new jobs, new cities, new cars, and other potentially stressful events.

When facing a stressor, you will benefit if you ask questions of people who do understand it; read about it; and take other actions to educate yourself about its nature and effects.

Coping self-statements. All people talk to themselves sometimes. Many people think that talking to yourself is a sign of craziness. Actually, the opposite may be more accurate: Not talking to yourself may be a sign of craziness. You may have noticed that you "talk yourself into" doing difficult things. Imagine taking your first

dive off a diving board or making your first public speech. You may recall making self-statements like, "C'mon, you can do it," "You know what to do," and "Go for it." These statements provide instructions and encouragements that help when facing challenges of all kinds.

Psychologists advise people facing such challenges to use four types of self-statements: preparing for the stressor, confronting and handling the stressor, coping with feelings at critical moments, and rewarding yourself for successful coping. The following lists provide examples of these four types of self-statements that you can use to manage almost any stressor. As you can see by the lists, people who use these self-statements actively cope with stressors. This approach encourages you to become a "hardy" coper in the same way that Suzanne Kobasa's hardy lawyers and executives manage stress. Both approaches to stress management encourage you to see stressors as opportunities to exert control and to enjoy and benefit from a challenge.

Think of a stressor that you faced recently. It could be taking an exam, going to a doctor or dentist, asking for a favor, or talking in front of a group of people. Try to imagine how you would talk yourself into and through these challenges. Then review the list of self-statements and see if you could have used some of them to help you manage that stressor.

Preparing for the stressor. Thoughts to use before the stressor occurs:

- What do I have to do?
- I can create a plan to deal with this.
- Thinking about what I have to do is certainly better than getting nervous about it.
- Worrying won't help. Plan.
- My anxiety tells me that I have a challenge facing me.
- I can learn from this.
- Just keep being logical and calm.

Confronting and handling the stressor. Thoughts to use during the stressor:

- I can handle this.
- I can meet this challenge.
- Just take it one step at a time; follow the plan.
- Beat the fear: Think of what I am doing.
- Relax. I'm in control. Just take a slow, deep breath.
- My tension just tells me to follow my plan; deal with this challenge.

Coping with feelings at critical moments. Thoughts to help control excess tension during the stressor:

- When tension comes, pause and breathe slowly.
- Focus on the present. Now, what do I have to do?
- I've handled this before and can manage it now.
- I'll rate my fear from one to ten and then watch it change.
- I'll just keep the tension manageable; I won't worry about eliminating it altogether.
- I can do this. It will be over in a certain amount of time.
- Okay, keep focused on what I want to do.
- This is not the worst thing that can happen.
- Remember, I don't have to handle this perfectly, just reasonably well.
- Focus on sensations to distract yourself: coldness, warmth, smells, touch, taste, sights, and sounds.
- Think about other times and places. Good feelings come with good thoughts.
- I'm in control.

Rewarding yourself for successful coping. Congratulate yourself for successful management of a difficult situation—after it's over:

- Nice going! I was able to do it.
- It wasn't as tough as I expected.
- Wait until I tell (a friend, spouse, other family member) about it.
- I'm making progress.
- My plan worked.
- I'm learning all the time.
- It's my thinking that creates tension. When I control my self-statements, I can control my tension.
- I'm doing better each time I use these self-statements.
- I'm really pleased with my progress.

Weight controllers face many stressors that can directly affect their efforts either to lose weight or maintain a low weight. For example, consider the impact of going to a party. Parties include lots of high-fat food, readily available alcoholic drinks, and people in a generally relaxed and unrestrained state. Some parties also go on late into the evening, increasing your feeling of tiredness. Parties also include people who might encourage you to eat or drink in problematic ways. How could you use the stress inoculation approach to handle this stressor?

First, the educational aspect of stress inoculation would encourage you to find out all you can about the event. The following are several questions asked by my clients (both to the party host and to themselves) to educate themselves about parties before going to them:

- How many people will be there?
- What kind of food will be served?
- More specifically, are there options for the main course and are there good options during the hors d'oeuvres or early phases of the party?
- Will there be people there with whom I would like to talk and spend time?
- Will I be bored?
- Will I be able to leave when I feel like it?

The answers to these questions determine whether the situation will create a major or minor challenge to your weight-control efforts. If low-fat options abound and if the people will provide good distractions, the situation will be easier to manage. On the other hand, a boring party combined with abundant high-fat food may require you to cope at a high level.

Coping self-statements can help you get through challenging parties. For example, you could try some of the following ideas:

Preparing:
I can create a plan that will get me through this.
I don't have to worry about this; I can plan for it.
I'm sure I can learn from this and get even better at managing these kinds of situations.
Plan:
1. Get a diet drink or a sparkling water and hang on to it.
2. Find the most interesting people available and talk with them.
3. Make a plan with my spouse to leave if I give him or her the signal.
4. Make the signal dramatic, if necessary—for instance, "We have to go now, dear!!!"

Confronting and handling:
I can handle this.
There are a lot of people here, but that gives me greater choices.
Stay focused and remember that "everything counts."

Coping at critical moments:
If I see some tempting morsel in the hors d'oeuvre phase, I'll grip my drink even more tightly.
Remember to find some low-fat alternatives; they've got to be here.
Even if I eat some problematic foods, I can still count it and record it.
Every food has finite calories and fat grams; nothing is going to kill me here.

Let me find somebody I can talk to who can make me laugh.

I can get something else to drink that will work.

Even if the main course is chock-full of problems, I don't have to eat a lot of it.

Reward myself for success:

Nice going. I basically followed the plan.

It was just a party and I handled it okay.

The plan was good even though I did eat a few things I didn't want to.

I think I'm getting better at this.

Some of my clients say that weight control requires a degree of obsessiveness. You have to concentrate intently when facing stressors, particularly stressors that can directly affect your weight-control efforts. If you can accept the requirement of this extra concentration, you can use it as a personal challenge. Stressors, demands from your life that can create negative tension, can also help you learn about yourself and help you become more of a master of your own fate.

Relaxation Techniques

The outline below shows some examples of "cued relaxation." This technique encourages you to include relaxation as part of your everyday life. By using the cues that you find in your normal environment to remind yourself to take a relaxation break, you can prevent little hassles from becoming big stressors.

Cued Relaxation

Instructions: Find some cues from your everyday life that you can use to remind yourself to take brief relaxation breaks. Such cues could include the ringing of your telephone, the drinking of water from a fountain, reaching for your wallet, or combing your hair. When the cue occurs, take a few seconds to use a relaxation technique.

Examples

Cue: phone call

1. Phone rings.
2. Answer the phone.
3. Use a breathing technique (e.g., slow rhythmic breathing).
4. During the call focus on breathing in a relaxed manner.
5. After the phone call, take another few seconds to execute the relaxation technique once again.

Cue: drinking water or coffee

1. Begin drinking.
2. Focus on the fluid and the sounds and sights of it.
   - What color is it?
   - What does it sound like specifically as you drink?
   - Concentrate on the texture of the fluid as it enters your mouth and goes down your throat.
3. Create a vivid image that involves water. For example:
   - You are on a beach in the summertime and you are watching a lake gently flow to the shore and retreat from the shore.
   - You are hiking on a mountain and you come upon a beautiful waterfall. You are watching the water flow and beat down on the rocks below. You are listening to the sounds and smelling the air.
4. Take a few minutes to stay in the image, keeping it vivid, using all of your senses to enliven the imagery.

Cue: reaching for your wallet

1. After your hand makes contact with the wallet, remind yourself to relax.
2. Tense and then relax some of the muscles in your hand and arm. Tense and relax those muscles at least twice.
3. Pay attention to the change in sensation from the tense to the relaxed state for each muscle group that you use. Focus on the

relaxed state for a few seconds and try to bring that sense of relaxation from the top of your head through your eyes and down to the rest of your body.

Thirty High-Risk Situations and Thirty Coping Responses

Some situations require more stress inoculation than others. Coping with these high-risk situations successfully can help you maintain momentum and prevent serious lapses. To identify which situations pose problems for you, read the following list of thirty high-risk situations.

Thirty High-Risk Situations

1. Getting home from work.
2. Friday night after work.
3. Watching TV.
4. Watching a movie in a theater.
5. Studying or reading at night.
6. Eating at your family's home (for example, at your parents' home).
7. Eating meals during the holidays (especially Halloween, Thanksgiving, Christmas, Hanukkah).
8. Being around someone who is encouraging you to eat something appealing that is high in fat and sugar.
9. Being in a bar, drinking alcoholic drinks.
10. Wanting to eat something when only high-calorie foods are available.
11. Seeing or smelling problematic foods.
12. Picnics.
13. Being at a party.
14. Eating in a favorite restaurant.
15. Attending business functions where food and drink are in abundance.

16. During coffee breaks.
17. When someone brings high-fat food into a meeting at your office (cookies, muffins, pizza).
18. Lunches with clients.
19. Being alone and/or feeling lonely.
20. When you feel blue, down, or depressed.
21. When you feel frustrated or angry.
22. When you are bored.
23. When you feel stressed or pressured.
24. When you are happy or relaxed.
25. After you have stuck to your weight-control plan for several days and feel like rewarding yourself for your hard work.
26. After you have lost several pounds and feel you deserve to take it easy.
27. After you have not stuck to your weight-control plan and think you have blown the program.
28. When you are hungry.
29. When you crave something specific (like steak, french fries, real ice cream, or Oreos).
30. After you had a particularly unsatisfying meal.

Can you think of other situations in which you struggle to cope? Do your high-risk situations change over time or do they change with the seasons? For example, some of my clients report wanting certain types of high-fat foods during the winter when they feel colder more often (e.g., ribs or meatloaf). Others say that the increased social activity during the summer, particularly picnics and other types of parties, can really get to them. See if you think the thirty coping responses listed below could help you.

Thirty Coping Responses

1. Leave the situation.
2. Call or talk to someone (for example, a friend, brother, sister).

3. Think about the reasons you want to control your weight and the benefits that will result from being thinner.

4. Exercise.

5. Do something enjoyable to distract yourself (for example, read a good book or magazine, visit a friend, listen to music, do a crossword puzzle, or see a movie).

6. Make your lunch and bring it with you.

7. Eat some low-calorie snacks that will fill you up (for example, carrots, celery, plain popcorn).

8. Drink a lot of water or other very low-calorie fluids (for example, noncaffeinated drinks such as diet soda, club soda with lemon or lime, bouillon, herbal tea).

9. Write an entry in a journal, diary, letter, or E-mail that allows you to express your feelings.

10. Reward yourself in ways other than eating food (for example, buy something inexpensive such as a tape, CD, or book; go somewhere pleasant like a movie, a friend's home, a park, or a sporting event; or do something else you enjoy like walking, dancing, or a favorite hobby).

11. Keep your home supplied with foods appropriate for your weight-control effort and eliminate foods you are trying to avoid or limit.

12. Shop for groceries on the weekend and cook meals for the coming week.

13. Keep a food diary.

14. Wait a half hour until the hunger or craving passes.

15. Forgive yourself. Controlling weight is very hard to do. When a slip or lapse happens, apply the brakes quickly and get back on track. A minor slip does not have to become a major disaster.

16. Remind yourself of all the negative consequences of being overweight.

17. Order lower-fat, lower-calorie foods.

18. Bring something you can eat with you (for example, low-calorie snacks for work; raw vegetables with a low-calorie dip to a party).

19. Do something to relax (for example, think of something pleasurable, take a shower or bath, or listen to soft music in a darkened room).

20. Suggest going to a place that offers appropriate food choices.

21. Tell yourself "Stop!" before you get swept away by the situation.

22. Meet your family or friends after they are out of the situation you find hard to handle.

23. Talk with a therapist, counselor, or religious or spiritual leader about high-risk situations and get their ideas about coping.

24. Focus on an image of yourself as a thinner and healthier person who controls his or her eating very effectively.

25. Become involved in after-work or weekend activities (for example, go to a concert or museum, do volunteer work).

26. Have soup before going to high-risk social or business functions.

27. Chew sugar-free gum.

28. Spray breath freshener in your mouth or brush your teeth.

29. Look at something that reminds you of your weight-control effort (for example, a colored dot placed on your watch or a picture of yourself as a thinner, healthier person).

30. Remind yourself that all food counts. Giving yourself permission because you've "blown it already today" just makes weight control more difficult.

Very High-Risk Situations

Three situations in particular give these coping responses a chance to show their stuff. Let's consider some specialized coping responses that you may find of use, in addition to the ones listed above, when handling the most universal of all high-risk situations: traveling, holidays, and restaurants.

Traveling

"When I go on my business trips to the East, I know exactly which places I like for meals and snacks. Unfortunately, most of the stuff is junk food. I know where the Pizza Huts are. I know where the Häagen-Dazs shops are. I even know where to get seemingly healthy but high-fat trail mixes. I seem drawn to these places when I travel. Somehow I convince myself that 'I need a break today. It's been a long frustrating day. It's okay to eat X, Y, Z.' "

Does this sound familiar? Traveling produces many frustrations and little control. We don't know if our plane is going to be late, where our luggage will wind up, and what food will be available at what time of the day. In addition, our usual patterns of eating are thrown to the wind by dehydration, jet lag, and changes in time zones. Many people also sleep less soundly when they travel. This produces yet another type of altered state. Disoriented by these strange internal states, we then have to face easily available high-fat, high-sugar foods—quite a combination!

Some of the problems when flying begin in the airplane itself. First, airplanes are kept extremely dry, as dry as the Sahara! It is critical that you drink at least one glass of noncaffeinated fluid for every hour you spend in flight. Consider bringing a bottle of water with you on the plane. This can improve your sense of control, while at the same time preventing dehydration. If you rely on flight attendants to get the fluid that you need and they are slow or unavailable, you may become both dehydrated and frustrated.

Another major problem that occurs when flying concerns the food. Remember, peanuts get 69 to 93 percent of their calories from fat, and a one-ounce packet contains 166 calories. That's a lot of fat and a lot of calories in one or two quick bites. Alcoholic drinks cause the body to lose water, exacerbating the already difficult fluid problem. In addition to their own calories, they also reduce restraint, which can pave the way for high-calorie eating and snacking.

The in-flight meals are perhaps the traveler's most notorious problem. Many of those small and sometimes very unappealing in-flight meals seem like snacks, but they often contain 600 or more calories, many of which come from fat. The boredom of flying makes these little unappetizing "snacks" seem much more appealing. And because many people think of these meals as snacks, they proceed to have a full meal soon after arriving at their destinations.

Special meals provide much healthier and tastier alternatives to standard in-flight meals. These special meals are just a phone call away. Most airlines require at least twenty-four hours' notice, but you can't beat the price. There is no extra charge for any of the special meals. Many more people are ordering special meals now than just a few years ago. However, less than 5 percent of travelers take advantage of this important opportunity. Special meals generally have about 33 percent fewer calories and much lower percentages of fat than the standard meals. For example, United Airlines serves about six thousand special meals per day, and their average special meal has less than 300 calories. These special meals include ones that meet religious specifications (kosher, Hindu, Moslem); meals for diabetics and vegetarians; low-calorie, low-cholesterol, and low-sodium meals; and seafood and fruit plates. That's quite a selection! I have found the seafood platter consistently good, often including crabmeat and other tasty and healthy food choices. Vegetarian meals also work well for some of my clients.

One way to increase the chances of your ordering these meals on time is to ask your travel agent to include a standing order for one of the special meals. This way when you book your flights, you book your meals at the same time.

Here are a few other travel tips for frequent fliers:

- If you did not order a special meal, try to minimize the fat in the standard meal. For example, as the flight attendant brings you the meal, hand back to him or her the margarine, salad dressing, and dessert. Simply give it to the attendant, making as minimal a comment as you like. You are not required to justify making healthy food choices if you do not wish to.
- Remove the skin from chicken and scrape away any gravies or sauces.
- Skip the eggs, omelets, sausages, and red-meat options. Instead, select cold cereal with fruit and skim milk for breakfast and eat chicken or pasta alternatives for other meals.
- Bring low-fat snack foods with you. Raisins, crackers, cereal, and pretzels may provide good alternatives to some of the snacks available. (The tricky part is to wait until you are in the air before munching.)
- Try to plan your meals carefully on the days that you travel. For example, if you've scheduled a lunch or a dinner meeting for when you arrive, consider turning down the in-flight meal or snack. This would be a good time to use your own low-calorie snack or request a special meal as an alternative.

Traveling by air presents many challenges, but so does traveling by car, bus, or train. All modes of travel create irregularities in schedules and moods. Many of my clients and I have found it particularly helpful to exercise in the morning before traveling. This provides some stress relief and makes it more tolerable to sit for hours.

Another key remedy for the travails of travel is planning. That is, by carefully (even obsessively) planning your traveling, you can avoid some of the common pitfalls. Weight controllers who plan their meals carefully and ensure that low-fat, low-calorie snacks are available, for example, take some of the risk out of traveling. Weight controllers who have reached the Acceptance stage often lose weight while traveling. They use traveling as an opportunity to seek out activity and to avoid the temptations of readily accessible refrigerators and cupboards.

Yet another challenge imposed by traveling concerns people. Consider the following story of Al's "Southern challenge," below.

Al's Southern Challenge

I am Jewish and I was born and raised in the City with Big Shoulders, Chicago. Emphasis on B-I-G. My wife grew up in Memphis, Tennessee, and she's Christian. Her parents, grandparents, and all of her relatives are from the South. That's really far south—emphasis on *south*. You could say we are from different worlds—because we are.

I've made huge changes in the way I eat and in the way I exercise. I've really been working at this for three and a half years now and I've lost 50 pounds. I still want to lose another 50, and I'm getting there. It's a struggle every day, but I'm getting there. My wife weighs 80 pounds less than I do and eats more food and calories every day than me. Most people find that hard to believe, but it's true. She eats desserts several times per week; I almost never do. She eats fried foods occasionally; I don't. I exercise all the time; she almost never does. It's just the biological breaks, I guess.

Well, this plays out in a pretty funny way when we go to visit her relatives in Tennessee. I don't think many of the people who live in the southern part of the United States have quite gotten into the low-fat-eating business. At least my wife's relatives sure haven't. They eat ham for practically every meal! Butter, biscuits, gravy, country ham, regular ham, mayonnaise, cakes, fried everything.

I've known these fine people for more than ten years now. I've just really confused them in the last three. They don't know how to feed me anymore, and it presents certain challenges for all of us. For example, after we get to my wife's aunt's house, which is where we sometimes stay for weekends when we visit,

I immediately go to the grocery store. I stock up on skim milk, fresh vegetables, no-salt pretzels, and a few other mainstays. They've learned that I just won't eat certain things. They've made a real effort to have raw vegetables available for me and to cook some foods that for them are unusual (like chicken instead of ham). They even go so far as to buy apples occasionally or some other snack food that I can eat. Unfortunately, the apples they buy don't quite meet my Chicago standards most of the time. They're usually rather anemic and bumpy. But it's a nice thought! They even avoid buttering and putting bacon fat on vegetables, quite a change for these people.

I make sure I exercise every day when I visit there. Sometimes this means getting up before my small children wake up, even if it's before the sun peeks out over the hills. This usually makes me tired, but it allows me to stay with the program in a difficult situation. Certainly these folks try to get me to eat and they sometimes make fun of me for my "strange ways." I try not to make a big deal out of it. We seem to have adjusted to each other reasonably well.

Al effectively asserted himself with his relatives. Family members can be food pushers. Food is a complex commodity; people use it to express themselves. Food can also be used to control situations and other people. Getting people to overeat helps some people feel less guilty about their own problematic habits. It is helpful to realize that traveling involves negotiating and asserting yourself with other people. The central question for you when you travel is: *Do you have the right to eat in a healthy, effective way wherever you are?* (The answer is *yes*).

Holidays

Thanksgiving is a classic holiday that many Americans consider a well-justified eating orgy. Actually, in the following Thanksgiving dinner menu, you can see that many of the elements of the classic Thanksgiving meal are healthy foods.

Food/Serving size	Calories
Turkey (no skin, half white meat, half dark meat), 3 oz.	148
Mashed potatoes, 1 cup	222
Gravy, ½ cup	61
Stuffing, ½ cup	250
Candied sweet potato, 1	144
Cranberry sauce, 2 Tbs.	52
Fresh fruit salad, ½ cup	62
Celery, 1 stalk	5
Carrot, ½	15
Bread, 1 roll	71
Butter, 1 pat	35
White wine, ½ cup	80
Pumpkin pie, 1 slice	300
Whipped cream, ¼ cup	200
Coffee	0
Total	**1,645**

The white-meat turkey without the skin, potatoes, fresh fruit salad, celery, carrots, and even the white wine pose no major problems. It's the stuffing, gravy, butter, pumpkin pie crust, and whipped cream that pile on the calories and the excess fat. The meal listed above derives 21 percent of its calories from fat. By selecting the low-fat components of the classic Thanksgiving dinner, you could have a perfectly satisfactory meal.

My colleagues and I have found that weight controllers who are focused and plan their Thanksgiving holiday usually cope with it quite well. First, the food is predictable. Second, the company and social aspects of the situation are predictable and possibly controllable. If you are serving the feast, you can invite people with whom you want to talk. If you are going somewhere, you can spend your time with the people who are interesting and enjoyable. Finally, Thanksgiving is also finite. It has a clear beginning and end. It doesn't go on and on and on for days and days with parties and parties and parties, the way Christmas does.

The Christmas season poses greater risks for weight controllers. Unlike Thanksgiving, Christmas lasts well beyond one particular day. There are pre-Christmas parties and minicelebrations. There are sugary "treats" at the office. There are rituals like baking Christmas cookies and other traditional high-fat, high-sugar foods. And, of course, this endless stream of parties can last for several weeks, right up through New Year's Eve. Alcohol also flows freely during this time of the year. Many restraints are lost and replaced instead by the "holiday spirit." All of this goes on during a time of the year when the coldness of the climate in many parts of the United States makes exercising especially challenging.

Easter and other holidays pose somewhat similar problems. These holidays also involve sugary and high-fat foods, they also last quite a while, and restraint often yields to the holiday spirit.

Not surprisingly, many people gain weight during the holiday season (from Thanksgiving through New Year's). Weight controllers may gain even more weight than the average person because of their biological predispositions toward weight gain. Weight controllers can also lose the positive momentum that they may have developed prior to the holiday season. Getting back into low-fat, low-sugar eating and intensive frequent exercising once you take a vacation from it is a major psychological challenge. I've seen many people become derailed during the holiday season and take months, sometimes years, to get back on track.

Successful weight controllers use several tricks of the trade during the holidays. Consider the following suggestions:

- *Plan ahead.* When you plan ahead, you can predict and control your world. For example, think about your next party. Who's going to be there and what kind of food will be served? You can call your host and get a preview of the menu. You can make a tentative list of what you will eat, with whom you will talk, and how you will stay focused. It is particularly important that you attempt to monitor your food record during the holiday season.

- *Avoid starvation before a celebration.* Starving before a big holiday meal can produce binge eating. Starving produces deprivation and a very strong biological response to the sight of food. This biological response includes the secretion of insulin and saliva. In other words, if you eat nothing or very little before a big holiday meal or party, you will get incredibly hungry. This reaction is more likely to lead to problematic eating than controlled eating. An alternative approach would include selecting low-fat, low-sugar foods for breakfast and lunch. Ironically, having a small snack just before leaving for the party may help as well.

- *Scope out the food scene.* After arriving, you can quickly survey the available options. Perhaps you will notice that there are fresh vegetables and other munchies that will work for you. You might also discover that the main course will keep you on a low-fat, low-sugar plan. This advance look may prevent you from eating high-fat snacks, such as chips, dips, nuts, and party mixes.

- *Use a food plan.* Once you are aware of the available and planned party foods, you can develop a specific food plan for what you will eat and a way of focusing on that plan. You can use a glass of diet soda or water to keep your attention on the conversation. You can also use this cue or some other cue (perhaps munching a raw vegetable) to remind yourself of your immediate goals and your long-range goals.

- *Refocus your holiday season.* This suggestion goes well beyond an individual event or party. Holidays are traditionally focused around food and celebrations. You can break that tradition. You can focus on other people, special projects, and finding new creative ways to relax. Some people develop their skills in winter sports; others focus on crackling fireplaces and reading some good books.

Restaurants

Americans ate 25 percent of their meals outside of their homes in 1975. In 2000, it is estimated that Americans will eat 50 percent of their meals outside of their homes. Restaurant meals account for almost 50 percent of every dollar Americans spend on food. Americans eat 25 percent of their restaurant meals at fast-food eateries, such as McDonald's, Burger King, Wendy's, and Pizza Hut.

You probably noticed that you, too, eat out more often now than ever before in your life. Restaurants offer the advantages of keeping you away from preparing food and the urge to nibble as you cook. On the other hand, restaurants often cook in mysterious ways, using more fat and more sugar than you would to prepare food. Some eateries can also lull you into making problematic food choices because of their style or atmosphere.

It requires clarity of thinking and assertiveness to eat healthfully in restaurants. It is your *right* to request that the food you order at a restaurant be prepared according to your wishes, so that you can get what you pay for. Most restaurateurs want to accommodate their patrons. In a recent survey conducted by MasterCard, more than 90 percent of the restaurateurs who were surveyed said they preferred hearing complaints about orders directly. They want you to be satisfied and to bring your business back to them. Still, some servers resist providing you with the information you want about food preparation. Remind yourself of your right to that information, then try making a polite request—even repeated requests, if necessary. This strategy should work well most of the time. For example:

Patron: "I'll take the chicken dish with broccoli and new potatoes. How is that prepared?"

Server: "How is what prepared?"

Patron: "The chicken."

Server: "I think it's broiled."

Patron: "In other words, it might be sautéed instead of broiled?"

Server: "Yeah."

Patron: "Could you check on that for me, please?"

Server: "Okay."

(Server leaves for two minutes to check on preparation of the chicken and then returns.)

Server: "It's broiled."

Patron: "Great. Then I'll go with the chicken. I'd like the vegetables grilled, with no butter added on them."

Server: "I don't think they put any butter on the vegetables or the potatoes."

Patron: "Please be sure that no butter or any sauces are added to the broccoli or the potatoes, okay?"

Server: "Okay."

Does this patron seem overly pushy to you? If you answered yes, you still have a problem. Remember, you have the right to get what you pay for. That includes knowing what you're getting. If your server does not comply with reasonable requests for this kind of information, you could ask to speak to the manager or the owner. You could also leave the restaurant. What does not work is to stay and eat foods that you want to avoid.

Sometimes my clients lament the limited choices in certain types of restaurants. One of my clients countered these laments eloquently. He said, "I can always find something to eat." He meant that he could always find something to eat that fits well with his weight-control program. Perhaps even he would be challenged by the notoriously limited menus in small-town bars, but for the most part his view coincides with that of virtually all successful weight controllers. Consider some of the options below for a variety of ethnic restaurants:

- *Cajun.* Seafood or vegetable gumbo or jambalaya (without sausage), grilled fish.
- *Chinese.* First ask, "What can you prepare without oil?" Stir-fries prepared with fat-free sauces, broths, or soy sauce are good choices; also chicken, seafood, and vegetables; soups (hot and sour, chicken, vegetable); chicken and shrimp dishes steamed without sauces.
- *French.* Poached, grilled, or steamed fish; chicken with wine sauce; Niçoise salads without oil.
- *Greek.* Chicken and fish shish kebabs; salads, couscous, rice.
- *Indian.* Tandoori chicken, prawns, fish.
- *Italian.* Pasta with red clam sauce, meatless marinara; pizza without cheese, with steamed vegetable toppings; minestrone soup (made without butter).
- *Japanese.* Sushi, chicken and fish teriyaki, tofu, and vegetables (avoid avocado, eel, mayonnaise, and mackerel).
- *Mexican.* Chicken and seafood enchiladas with no cheese; tamales with no cheese; chicken or shrimp fajitas (without sour cream or guacamole), made with "as little oil as possible"; chicken taco salad (no cheese); salsa (request tortillas as a side dish and dip them, instead of chips, into the salsa).
- *Thai.* First ask, "What can you prepare without oil?" Then, stir-fried shrimp, chicken, and vegetable dishes can work for you. Also, soups, especially sweet and sour (tom yum) soup; chicken and cucumber salads.

A critical saying to remember when ordering food in restaurants is:

If you don't know what the food is or how it was prepared, assume the worst!

This means that you can assume more oil or fat of some kind is added if you are not sure that the food is safe. This saying directs you to find something on the menu that you can rely on. If you look diligently enough, on virtually every menu you, too, "can always find something to eat."

> "[People] are disturbed not by things, but by the view which they take of them."
>
> —Epictetus, *The Enchiridion,* first century A.D.

> "There's nothing either good or bad but thinking makes it so."
>
> —William Shakespeare, *Hamlet*

S E V E N

❖

Maintaining Success

Truth #9: Maintaining weight loss is actually easier, *not* harder, than losing weight.

Alice Still Lives Here

Alice turned forty-eight today. True enough, forty-eight isn't one of those supposedly especially important birthdays (like forty or fifty), but on her birthdays she's often taken stock of where she's been and where she's going—whether she was supposed to or not.

Alice mentioned that she and I have been meeting every week for more than four years now. She recalled her initial enthusiasm for the work we did together and how it helped her harness a lot of energy for weight control. Alice recorded every morsel of food that she ate for many, many months in a row back then. Her energized focusing helped her lose more than 40 pounds from her five-foot-six (and initially 240-pound) body in those first six months.

After that initial Honeymoon, the struggles became more like swamps. Troubles at work, the constant and crazy-making strain of living alone, and other aspects of everyday life began to overtake her efforts to exercise, monitor her eating, and stay focused and optimistic. "But," she said, "I never gave up. I came up with new plans almost every week (sometimes almost every day). Sometimes my plans would include new ways of exercising. Can you remember all of the different classes and clubs I joined? Sometimes my plans would stress different types of foods—like my soup plan or my vegetarian plan. I tried Optifast [a liquid meal-replacement approach] about fifteen different times over these years: Sometimes it helped me lose weight, sometimes the change inspired renewed efforts, sometimes it was just another frustration. But I never gave up, and I never will! I may not get to where I was thirty years ago, but I am stronger now, healthier, and much thinner than I would be if I did not stay with the struggle every day.

"I'm learning to live with the struggle. The struggle, and living with it, is okay. At least most of the time it's okay. It's become my roommate! We don't always get along, but we find a way to stay together. It's where I live." Alice now weighs 60 pounds less and is quite physically fit compared to the way she was when she first walked into my office more than four years ago.

The Basic Plan: Persistence

Like Alice, all successful weight controllers persist. They persist in spite of their bodies' seemingly insatiable desire to eat. They exercise despite the usual excuses of time, effort, money, and aches and pains. They persist even though they live in the age of cheese fries and six-cup pasta entrées. They even persist after a vacation full of deviations or a holiday full of unresisted temptations, and after several very, very unwanted pounds have returned—yet again.

The Choice of Acceptance

Have you generally reached the Acceptance stage of successful weight control? You may recall from chapter 2 that in this stage, people settle in for the long haul. They experience a *peaceful sense of resolve* about weight control. They feel comfortable and have a clear direction for handling their challenging biologies. They also

refine their knowledge of nutrition in this stage. Their understanding of the factors that affect weight control becomes clear as
well. They do struggle with their focusing or commitment sometimes. This happens quite often when they go on vacations or when
their schedules are disrupted by illness or travel. If you are in this
stage, you now view exercise as either enjoyable or at least acceptable. You exercise very consistently. You also consistently monitor
your food and exercise. You actually prefer food to be prepared in a
healthy way, and you are willing to assert yourself effectively in
restaurants and other social situations to ensure that your food
works for you. Another way of thinking about this assertiveness is
the term "aggressive self-protectiveness." If this term applies to you,
you feel both confident and very willing to protect yourself against
situations or other people that challenge your weight-control efforts.
You are unwilling to place yourself in a position where you would be
"mindless" again about your eating, exercising, and weight. You have
made a very active choice to pursue the life of a successful weight
controller.

A Four-Step Insurance Policy

What is your plan to keep your eating, exercising, coping, and
focusing skills sharp and consistent? What would you do, for example,
if you found yourself eight pounds heavier than your usual weight?
Consider adopting some version of the following four steps to
ensure that you stay within the boundaries of an effective weight-
control program:

Step 1. Self-directed change: Taking your best shot. This may
include adopting a low-fat eating plan such as the "Almost Never"
plan or the Popcorn Plan.

Step 2. Get a little help from your friends. If Step 1 does not produce positive results within a few weeks, you can involve others in
your exercising program or your eating plan. Commitments are
strengthened when they become more public.

Step 3. Get help from others with the same problem. Both Take Off Pounds Sensibly (TOPS) and Weight Watchers can help some people, some of the time.

Step 4. Get help from professionals. Hospitals and medical centers sometimes offer programs, such as Optifast, that can help more people more of the time than the nonprofessional programs listed in Step 3. Look for programs conducted by psychologists with expertise in cognitive-behavior therapy. Programs that provide help for unlimited periods of time (no less than one year) are especially worthy of consideration. Calls to local hospitals and to the psychology departments of local colleges and universities may prove helpful. The following two national organizations have listings of psychologists in virtually every area of the United States: Association for Advancement of Behavior Therapy (212 279-7970) and American Psychological Association (202 336-5500).

The critical aspect of persistence in weight control is finding a way to nurture your commitment to it. This can occur only if you maintain practices such as weighing yourself at least weekly. Another aspect of commitment pertains to clothing. If your clothes get tighter, consider taking the necessary steps to activate the long-term plan. Simply having clothes enlarged or buying larger clothes can deactivate your plan and diminish your commitment.

Maintaining Hope

Keeping your commitment alive means keeping hope alive. How do you do that consistently, despite the setbacks of everyday life? Three psychological techniques have helped thousands of weight controllers breathe life into a sagging sense of hope: reattribution technique, rational emotive techniques, and assertiveness training. The following sections consider each of these approaches and help you see how to use them to maintain your success.

Reattribution Technique

Attributions are beliefs about the causes of behavior. These beliefs decide or contribute responsibility for actions or thoughts. The reattribution technique involves changing your attributions about problems in your weight-control program into hopeful ways of thinking about them.

Attributions have three dimensions:

Internal-External
Stable-Unstable
Global-Specific

Internal attributions assign causes of events to yourself. *External attributions* assign causes to others or the environment. For example, what if someone who was trying to change her eating and exercising habits ate several handfuls of peanuts and two desserts at a party. She could blame herself exclusively for the problem ("I am just very weak and I don't want to change"). Or she could decide that the party was a "high-risk situation" that she did not manage effectively. Viewing the party as a problematic situation places some of the blame for the problem on the environment. This is an external attribution.

Stable attributions are those that assert that causes remain consistent over time. If you gained weight last week, you could decide that you just don't have the willpower to lose weight, or you could believe that you do not really care about losing weight. When you use *unstable attributions* when thinking about the causes of weight gain, you are deciding that change will occur. These unstable attributions can help you feel more hopeful. For example, "I had a particularly stressful week; I could have focused on planning and exercising more thoroughly than I did last week."

Global attributions assign responsibilities for behaviors and events in very general terms. For example, let us imagine that you worked hard at weight control all week and then did not lose any weight. You could decide that your weight stayed the same because "life isn't fair" or "that is just the way it goes sometimes." These are very general beliefs about the causes of your problem. More *specific attributions* include "The scale is an imperfect measure of change" or "Perhaps I did not exercise as much as I thought I did" or "Perhaps I ate more than I thought I did."

The most helpful attributions are those that keep you hopeful. Therefore, when you are making good progress toward changes in eating and exercising (and weight loss), try to attribute that progress to yourself (internal attribution). It also helps to avoid making internal, stable, and global attributions for problems or lapses. If you believe that something within you that you cannot change causes you problems, you will certainly increase your chances of failure. *When you encounter problems, try to find the* external *factors that contributed to them.* Work toward realizing that the causes of the problem are *specific* factors that can change. Remember, this reattribution technique does not simply rationalize or blindly explain away problems. It helps you stay hopeful by encouraging you to view problems in perspective.

Rational Emotive Techniques (RET)
Here are some common irrational beliefs:

- A person should be loved, or approved of, by almost everyone.
- In order to be worthwhile, a person should be competent in almost all respects.
- Things should always be exactly the way I want them to be; it's terrible when they're not.
- Every problem has (should have, must have) an ideal solution; it is catastrophic when the solution is not found.

If you believe these statements and live by them, you will undoubtedly become anxious or depressed quite often. Psychologist

Albert Ellis developed the idea that accepting irrational beliefs as ultimate truths can create unpleasant emotions. You can recognize the irrational beliefs by the language used when stating them. In the examples above, several statements include the words "should" and "must." These terms limit our choices. These terms are "absolutisms" or "categorical imperatives." When you tell yourself you "have to," "should," and "ought to" do something, you tell yourself that you have very few choices. The more rules you force yourself to follow, the less freedom you experience. Almost everyone rebels against restrictions in their freedom. The experience of restricted freedom is highly stressful.

Other words that suggest irrational thinking include *all*, *always*, *awful*, *essential*, *every*, *horrible*, *terrible*, and *totally*. These words *exaggerate* problems or concerns. Such exaggerations contribute to a feeling of hopelessness. You may recall an earlier discussion emphasizing the importance of active problem solving for maintaining weight change. Using language and beliefs that encourage hopelessness leads to giving up.

When you recognize yourself using absolutisms or exaggerations, you can dispute these irrational beliefs. Consider the following examples of irrational beliefs and the disputing responses that can modify them and renew your hopefulness.

Irrational Beliefs	Disputing Responses (Counterarguments)
I'll never be able to lose all of this weight.	I've got to begin somewhere. I can start by focusing on the first five pounds. If I don't try, I'll probably continue to gain weight and feel worse about it.

Irrational Beliefs	Disputing Responses (Counterarguments)
I look awful. I can never lose enough weight to look decent.	It doesn't help to "awfulize." Certainly people don't stop in the street and faint because of my looks. I look okay. I'm just overweight, and that creates problems for me. Other people have been successful in losing weight, so why can't I? If I take it one step at a time, I can get there.
I've lost eight pounds and no one has even noticed.	Probably someone has noticed, even if they haven't said something to me. Commenting on someone's weight loss can be rude. Some people say things like "You look so much better!" That implies that you looked lousy before losing the weight. I've noticed the weight loss and can feel it in my clothes and my energy level. That's as important as anything.
I have to lose weight fast.	Of course, I would prefer to lose weight quickly. Who wouldn't? But if I lose weight slowly and steadily, I'll still get to where I want to be. I haven't exercised much for the last several years, and my eating has included too much fat and too much sugar. It

Irrational Beliefs	Disputing Responses (Counterarguments)
	took a long time for this pattern to develop and it will take a while to change it.
I'll gain back all the weight I have lost and then some.	Managing weight is very challenging. I'm still learning to manage my weight, and lapses from time to time are typical. I can expect some fluctuations in weight. That does not mean I will ultimately be unsuccessful. It makes very little sense to predict failure when the future is not known to anyone.
I'm afraid that others will see me as a failure.	Not everyone is concerned about my weight. Many people can respect how hard I try. Being overly concerned with others' opinions of me is a burden I don't want. I can choose to ignore what others say and appreciate what I accomplish.
I'm afraid I won't like myself after I've lost the weight.	Making arbitrary, negative predictions about the future won't benefit me. I am much more than my weight. There are many things I like about myself. I can feel good about my success and my improved health by staying on track.

202 ❖ *The 9 Truths about Weight Loss*

Irrational Beliefs	Disputing Responses (Counterarguments)
I can't stand it when people compliment me.	I really *can* stand it. I just don't enjoy it. Some people who offer compliments recognize the hard work required to lose weight. I don't have to think of their remarks as a pressure or burden. I can decide to what extent I will pressure myself to manage my weight.
It's absolutely impossible for me to resist these cookies. I really love them.	How can I love a cookie? A cookie is butter and sugar and flavorings. It's not a person, and "loving it" just gets in my way. It is certainly possible for me to resist these cookies. If someone offered me a million dollars to give up these cookies for the rest of my life, I wouldn't eat these cookies. I can do it for myself as well as for some make-believe reward. I have the power to resist eating anything I want to.
I can't stand being a fanatic every day of my life.	First of all, I can stand it. Second of all, no one says I must do everything every single day. I can back off some days and be more aggressive on others.
I shouldn't be concerned about what others think of me.	Humans are social creatures. It's reasonable for me to be

Irrational Beliefs	Disputing Responses (Counterarguments)
	concerned about the opinions of others. It's unreasonable for me to think that I live my life solely based on the opinions of others. I can make choices about how I look, how I exercise, and almost all other aspects of my life.
I shouldn't have eaten that brownie.	Eating high-fat and high-sugar foods is problematic. It would be better if I didn't eat the brownie. However, I don't want to force myself to live with arbitrary rules ("shoulds"). If I eat a problematic food, I can monitor it and think of it as a problem to be solved.

You can see the use of exaggerations and absolutisms in this listing of irrational beliefs. Another method of categorizing irrational beliefs uses words and phrases to define different types of irrational thinking. The list below shows the definitions of seven types of irrational thinking. When you find yourself grappling with these irrational beliefs, try arguing with yourself. Dispute the absolutisms and exaggerations. You'll find yourself feeling better, more optimistic, and not at all hopeless.

Seven Types of Irrational Beliefs

1. *Arbitrary inference:* Drawing a conclusion when evidence does not support the conclusion or is lacking entirely. "Since I didn't lose weight last week, I must be fooling myself to think I'm trying."

2. *Overgeneralization:* Creating a general rule from a single incident or observation. "I didn't walk very far today; I can't be serious about losing weight."

3. *Catastrophizing or magnification:* Exaggerating a problem or an event to make it seem hopeless or impossible to change. "I didn't lose weight last year; I can't do this."

4. *Cognitive deficiency:* Disregarding a relevant event or situation. "I know I ate a whole pizza last week, but I still can't believe I didn't lose weight."

5. *Dichotomous reasoning:* Believing that there are only two sides to an issue (good / bad, right / wrong) and no in-betweens. "I am either on a diet or off it."

6. *Oversocialization:* Failing to recognize and challenge the arbitrariness of many cultural mores. "I need liposuction to lose weight and a nose job to look decent. You can't be too thin."

7. *Negative thinking:* Focusing on aspects of behavior that you want to decrease and virtually excluding more positive thoughts. "I didn't exercise on three of seven days this week."

Assertiveness Training

Can you recall your reaction to being put down or taken advantage of or in some way interpersonally squashed or squelched? Frustrated, angry, anxious, and depressed feelings often follow such experiences. Expressing yourself openly, honestly, directly, and clearly can prevent those unpleasant emotional effects. This type of communication lets others know you are a person who has rights—including the right to be treated kindly and respectfully.

Assertiveness is defined as any act that serves to maintain a person's rights; it is the open expression of preferences by words or actions in a manner that causes others to take them into account. When someone attempts to take advantage of you or treats you disrespectfully, you can react *assertively*, *aggressively*, or *unassertively*. *Assertive* behavior enhances your sense of self. It is expressive and it helps you feel good about yourself. It may or may not achieve the desired goal, however. *Aggressiveness,* by contrast, usually achieves desired goals by hurting or taking advantage of others. Aggressiveness is also expressive, but at the expense of other people. *Unassertive* behavior involves preventing yourself from standing up for your own rights. It often produces hurt, anxious, and angry feelings. It certainly fails to accomplish the goal of standing up for your rights.

An example of potential violations of your rights that concern weight controllers is ordering a meal prepared in a low-fat way in a restaurant and having the server refuse to comply with your wishes. You certainly have the right to get what you pay for. Agreements at home with family members also rely on respectful treatment. If your spouse agrees to eat potato chips and candy outside of the house, you can justifiably become concerned when Milky Ways or M&Ms invade your kitchen cabinets. These situations sometimes lead to loud conflicts. Aggressive demands for change, when met with resistance, produce interpersonal fireworks. An assertive approach is kinder and gentler. It states concerns directly and makes specific requests for change. It provides a choice to the other person. The person may or may not respond in a desired fashion.

Listed below are seven key aspects of assertiveness. If you are going to assert yourself, it helps to know how to use all seven elements. Consider the example of the invasion of the junk food. Let's say the weight controller and spouse had agreed to ban such food from their house. The weight controller could angrily protest this "gross violation of our agreement." Resistance and hostility might flow from this exchange. In contrast, consider the likely reaction to "Honey, I really have to struggle to control my eating. You recognized this six months ago when you agreed to ban junk food in the house. It upsets me to have this agreement violated. I would really appreciate it if you would get rid of the candy and chips tonight." Try delivering a message like this directly and forcefully, with appropriate eye contact and body language. Your spouse will not feel attacked. He or she might help you stay focused and enthusiastic. Your spouse may not comply with your request; however, he or she will probably remember the agreement and abide by it in the future. In any case, a loud, angry argument will almost certainly not emerge from this assertion.

Seven Elements of Assertiveness

- *Eye contact.* Looking directly at another person when you are speaking to him or her. This effectively declares that you are sincere about what you are saying.
- *Body posture.* The "weight" of your messages to others will be increased if you face the person, stand or sit appropriately close to him or her, lean toward him or her, and hold your head erect.
- *Gestures.* A message accented with appropriate gestures takes on an added emphasis. Overenthusiastic gesturing, however, can be distracting.
- *Facial expression.* Ever see someone trying to express anger while smiling or laughing? It just doesn't come across. Effective assertions require an expression that agrees with the message.
- *Voice tone, inflection, volume.* A whispered monotone will hardly convince another person that you mean business. A shouted epithet will bring a person's defenses into the path of communication. A level, well-modulated conversational statement can prove convincing without intimidating.
- *Timing.* Make spontaneous expression your goal. Hesitation may diminish the effect of an assertion. Judgment is necessary, however, to select an appropriate occasion. For example,

speaking to your boss in front of a group of his or her subordinates may decrease his or her responsiveness to your request. Requesting a few quiet moments in a private office can promote acceptance of your assertion.

- *Content.* I saved this obvious dimension of assertiveness for last. Although *what* you say is clearly important, it is often less important than most people believe. A fundamental honesty in communication works best. That may mean saying forcefully, "I'm damn mad about what you just did!" rather than "You're an S.O.B.!" People who have, for years, hesitated because they "didn't know *what* to say" have found that the practice of saying *something* to express their feeling at the time helps them communicate more effectively.

Sometimes assertiveness in restaurants can prove quite challenging. The account below presents a particularly famous, and funny, example of assertiveness, under duress, at a restaurant. Although it might not have helped Jack Nicholson's character, some weight controllers find it easier to assert themselves in restaurants when they order first among a group of people. When you order first, you may get more of the server's attention and find yourself less tempted by the higher-fat orders of your friends.

The World's Most Famous Order of Wheat Toast

"I'd like some wheat toast, please," said Jack Nicholson's Bob Dupea in the movie *Five Easy Pieces.*

"Sir, you can only order what's on the menu," responded the waitress in the roadside diner.

"I don't understand. Do you have wheat bread?" replied Bob Dupea.

"Yeah," responded the waitress.

"Do you have a toaster?" asked Dupea.

"Yeah," answered the waitress.

"Then why can't you put the wheat bread in the toaster and make wheat toast?" inquired Dupea.

"Like I said before, you can only order what's on the menu," the waitress answered rather sternly.

"Okay, I'll make it as easy for you as I can. I'd like . . . a chicken salad sandwich on wheat toast. No mayonnaise, no butter, no lettuce," said Dupea.

"A number two," the waitress called out. "Chicken sal san. Hold the butter, the lettuce, and the mayo. . . . Anything else?"

"Yeah," he answered. "Now all you have to do is hold the chicken, bring me the toast, give me a check for the chicken salad sandwich, and you haven't broken any rules!"

Managing Your Environment

In *Five Easy Pieces*, the character played by Jack Nicholson found himself in an environment that was antagonistic to ordering a simple serving of toast. Part of the Acceptance phase of successful weight control involves taking steps so that your environment supports your efforts. You want to cultivate an aggressive stance, a self-protective attitude toward your world to allow you to maintain your approach to weight control forever. One of the most powerful ways to do this is to arrange the world within which you live so that it supports and promotes effective weight control. In this section, several ideas that successful weight controllers frequently use show you how to build momentum for the long haul by keeping your environment safe and encouraging of your efforts.

Stimulus Control

Stimulus control refers to the ability of certain situations or stimuli to control behavior. This means that certain situations can affect eating or exercising patterns in a direction that is either positive or negative. For example, when you see a commercial on television for fast-food hamburgers, you may feel particularly hungry and head toward the refrigerator. This means that watching television can actually become a stimulus for eating.

Another example of stimulus control concerns the places where you eat. People who eat while driving around in a car or in a bus are more likely to eat in many different situations than people who eat only in their kitchens or dining rooms. Some people eat when they are preparing food. For these individuals, the stimulus of preparing food affects their eating. Another example is the clock. When the clock strikes twelve, many people experience a strong desire to eat. The features of the environment such as the time of day, other people eating, food advertisements, and even the sight of food often affect overweight people more than nonoverweight people.

The following suggestions use the principle of stimulus control to reduce the number of stimuli that will encourage you to eat:

- *Decrease the number of eating situations.* Attempt to limit the number of situations in which you allow yourself to eat. Try to focus your eating primarily in kitchens, dining rooms, and restaurants. Avoid eating in family rooms, living rooms, or while watching television. If you do allow yourself to eat while watching television or in the movies, try to limit the type of eating. Perhaps you can allow yourself to eat only low-fat popcorn or fat-free pretzels in these circumstances. Also be aware that eating at your desk or while working at a computer can create stimulus-control problems.
- *Place food only in food areas.* It is best to keep all the food in your house in food areas. Having food available in candy dishes or glove compartments of cars just causes more interest in eating than you need. If you avoid keeping or bringing food to

your room for nighttime eating and snacking, you will also feel less hungry.

- *Discontinue noneating activities in food areas.* In food areas such as kitchens and dining rooms, it would be helpful if you primarily stored, prepared, or ate food there. Sometimes people work or sew or talk while sitting around kitchen or dining room tables. Try to avoid placing yourself in those situations. Food areas are associated with eating. If you put yourself in those areas frequently, you will stimulate your appetite. This makes it more difficult to avoid eating at times when you are trying to do other things.

- *Make eating a "pure experience."* Besides storing all food in one area and excluding noneating activities from that area, it is helpful to make eating a pure experience. In other words, it may help you reduce the amount that you eat if you engage in no other activity other than consuming food while you eat. For instance, try to avoid watching television, listening to the radio, reading newspapers, or doing schoolwork while you are eating. You may, of course, talk with family or friends while eating, but try to avoid staying at the table after you finish eating. While you are eating, try to concentrate as much as possible on the taste, texture, and smell of the food. You may find that you enjoy eating more by focusing on the "pure experience" of eating rather than on all of the other activities associated with eating. For people who live alone, eating with fewer or different kinds of stimulation can make eating a pure experience. Many people who live alone eat while watching television or reading. Try eating without television if you live alone, at least occasionally. Perhaps you will notice less "mindless" eating when you do this.

Support for Stimulus Control

The account below shows the challenges to spouses and other family members that the quest for stimulus control can create. How can you find a balance between creating an ideal or safe eating environment and allowing your family its treats?

Marge: Keeping Home Sweet Home Safe

Marge and her husband, Mike, have an excellent relationship. They work and play together and have a wonderful daughter. They are both successful professionals, and they respect each other's abilities and talents.

Marge has a substantial weight problem. She began the program with me several years ago. At that time she weighed 220 pounds (she is five foot two). She locked into a remarkably long Honeymoon stage and lost weight very steadily for more than a year. She exercised fanatically and added weight training to her treadmill work, StairMaster sessions, and walking. She relied on frozen foods, pasta, and potatoes as her mainstays. After about one and a half years, she reached her weight goal (140 pounds). She diligently monitored all of her food intake and her exercise output. Marge handled a variety of tensions effectively and received a lot of support from Mike. While she was in the Honeymoon stage, nothing Mike did or ate had any real effect on her. Unfortunately, Honeymoon stages do not last forever. After some major conflicts at work, Marge had to change jobs in a difficult situation, and her eating and exercising became less of a priority in her life. She began regaining weight and getting into binge eating occasionally.

During this Frustration stage, Mike's eating habits began to have negative effects on Marge. Mike never had a weight problem and could eat almost anything he wanted to without gaining weight. He frequently ate potato chips, M&Ms, and a variety of high-fat foods. When he and Marge watched the news or a movie at night, instead of munching on air-popped popcorn (as she did consistently during the Honeymoon stage), Marge began nibbling on Mike's high-calorie snacks. Once she opened that door, she found it hard to close. In other words, once she began eating potato chips instead of air-popped popcorn, the popcorn seemed like "cardboard" and she found the high-fat snacks "almost irresistible."

I encouraged Marge to bring Mike in for a meeting with me. The three of us discussed how Marge's problem was like a chronic disease. If Marge had a heart condition, cancer, or diabetes, Mike would have no problem making some adjustments in his life to keep Marge healthy. He had more trouble with this issue because he felt that he had a right to eat the way he wanted. We discussed this concern and concluded that Mike's freedom required some modification to help his wife stay healthy. He agreed to accommodate Marge and to keep all high-fat snacks out of the house. Marge found that it was much easier for her to exhibit self-control when her environment was well-controlled. Her Frustration stage became an Acceptance stage. She no longer snacked on high-fat foods and began getting back to her goal weight. During the past year, she has maintained a very good weight for her (approximately 150 pounds).

The story of Marge and Mike raises some important points. People sometimes think that good self-control means being able to stare at a chocolate cake five inches from your face and resist eating it. A much better form of self-control involves keeping the chocolate cake away from your face. In other words, self-control also means managing your environment to promote healthy behaviors. Marge learned that her self-control was dependent on keeping her home safe. For Marge, it meant a home in which no high-fat snacks were available.

This applies to most weight controllers. It requires some adjustment by families of weight controllers to live like this. High-fat snacks do not help anyone have a better life. However, our culture views these snacks as important fun treats. Some people feel deprived and angry if they cannot have them. Weight controllers often try to convince their families to help them take care of themselves by keeping these foods away from their homes. Remember, weight controllers have much greater biological responses to the sight, and perhaps even the thought, of some of these very tempting foods. Is it fair or reasonable for families of individuals who have this biological handicap to challenge their handicap every day? Families could accommodate their weight controllers by eating high-fat foods outside of the home. Is that too much to ask?

The best way for weight controllers to encourage their families to make this transition is to ask them to take an understanding approach. Some weight controllers create difficulties when they try to change their family's eating patterns overnight. Asserting "It's time for us to get rid of all of this junk food—now!" promotes resentment and anger. You could simply ask your family to understand the biological challenge you face.

Consider using something like the following approach to make your home a safe home: "I really need your help. My biology responds very dramatically to the sight and smell of high-fat foods. This makes it much more difficult for me to control my eating. If I have trouble controlling my eating, I don't feel good and I won't stay healthy and satisfied with myself. Because of this, I would really like your help to keep certain foods out of our house. I know this is a sacrifice for you, but please consider doing it for me." The exact wording makes no difference. The approach of asking for help, rather than demanding it, can make all of the difference. Should cookies or potato chips appear, try a gentle reminder.

Slumps and Slump Busters

You can develop the most remarkable and consistent skills at maintaining hope and managing your environment. You can generally feel hopeful and live in a perfectly safe place (in terms of food). Yet virtually all weight controllers will suffer slumps. Your weight loss stalls or reverses, and your spirits follow suit. Let's consider some of the major causes of these slumps and then discuss several ideas that you can use to break such unfortunate trends.

Lapse versus Relapse

One of my most successful clients, Nancy, had lost 60 pounds, getting to an excellent weight for her. Then she took a memorable trip to Mexico. She came to a realization about the nature of relapses in the weight-control effort. Take a look at Nancy's story and see if you can identify what helped her reorient her thinking.

Nancy's Realization: "No One Promised Me That Life Was Fair."

I went on vacation to Mexico and it was as if I had never heard of weight control. I just ate what I felt like, laid around in the sun, and had a great time. Maybe it was being in a different country, where everything was different. Somehow I just forgot who I was and what my body was about.

I came back after two relaxing weeks and stared at that metal monster in my bathroom. It took me two days to get back on it, but finally I did. I had gained eight pounds! I couldn't believe it! It's just not fair. It took me a while, but I realized that no one ever promised me that life was fair. I remembered what I had learned about the biological aspects of weight problems. I realized that my fat cells "never go on vacation." That's not fair; that's just the way it is.

I got back into monitoring my eating, and I got back out there and started walking every day again. The weight started to come back down. It took me two months (of hard labor) to get back to where I was before that vacation. I'm hoping the lesson in this is to find a way of relaxing without ignoring what my body is about.

The biology of excess weight makes it *impossible* for anyone to eat perfectly. Those hungry fat cells and associated hormones make an occasional french fry or doughnut virtually irresistible. Since perfection in eating is impossible, occasional lapses occur for even the most persistent weight controllers.

A *lapse* is a temporary problem. A lapse is a temporary detour from the overall plan. Lapsing does not have to lead to relapsing. A *relapse* is a full-blown change back into old, problematic styles of behavior.

Successful weight controllers persist in the face of the inevitable lapses. They realize that an occasional doughnut or ice cream cone is simply a problem, not a catastrophe. They view these deviations as acceptable, not earthshaking. Lapses begin becoming relapses when you discontinue monitoring your eating and exercising. If you eat four pieces of pizza and consider it a disaster, you may give up monitoring for that day, for that week, or for that year. If you eat the pizza and consider it a problem to be solved, you will write it down, calculate its calories and fat grams, and try to understand how you could have prevented that problem from occurring.

Nancy prevented her rather major lapse from becoming a full-blown relapse. More minor and usual lapses occur when people eat occasional high-fat or high-sugar foods. To prevent lapses from turning into relapses, remember two things:

- Lapses are inevitable.
- Lapses won't become relapses if you maintain your self-monitoring.

After you experience the inevitable lapse, try to write it down and deal with it as a problem to be solved. Figure out what led to the lapse, forgive yourself for lapsing, and move on from there. Take a look at the stories below and what can happen when lapses turn into relapses.

When Lapses Become Relapses:
Three Weight Controllers' Stories

· ·

Anna's Dangerous Doughnut

- "I had lost 42 pounds. It was quite a struggle. It took me almost a year of hard labor. Then there was this doughnut! I had been feeling so good, getting into some old clothes, and I just ate this doughnut. I figured, 'I've got this thing controlled. I can eat a doughnut.' The doughnut led to other problem foods like muffins. I started eating ice cream (full-fat) again, also. For some reason, I stopped exercising. It had taken me almost a year to lose the 42 pounds, but only a couple of months to regain it all, and then some."

Jeanne's Comfort Foods

- "I joined the Optifast program. I ate nothing but the powder for twelve weeks and lost almost 50 pounds. I exercised practically everyday (mainly walking). I kept participating in maintenance groups for three and a half months after the initial fast. I lost another 5 pounds during that period. My relationship with my husband had never been the greatest. We started having more bitter fights toward the end of the fast. Sometimes we would fight and scream at each other and other times we would be walking around each other in stony silence. We separated about the same time I discontinued participating in the maintenance groups in the Optifast program. Food became a reliable source of comfort again. Instead of watching every fat gram I ate, I just let myself eat what I felt like eating. It didn't take me long to regain the weight."

Jeff's Broken Leg, Broken Program

- "I joined a professional weight-control program two years ago. I was a fanatic. I ate between 600 and 800 calories a day and exercised every day. I had to start out slowly because I was 120 pounds overweight. I started walking and then I graduated to fast walking and weight training. I bought a treadmill and a

StairMaster and turned my den into a minigym. I was determined to beat this thing! Somehow I managed to stay on this intensely focused program for over a year. I lost 110 pounds and was feeling really good. Then I broke my leg in a skiing accident. It was a hairline fracture, but it was enough to sideline my exercise for two months. I was frustrated and began losing focus. I discontinued my involvement in the program and stopped monitoring my eating and exercising. After the two-month layoff was over, I tried getting myself to walk again. It was painful, and I had trouble staying with it. It would have been helpful for me to rejoin my program. I finally did that last week, after regaining 95 of the 110 pounds that I had lost. It's painful to face myself. I tried making it on my own and I couldn't do it. I know I can get back into this again, and this time I'm never going to quit it."

Managing Injuries and Illnesses

Momentum is a magical thing. In weight control, you can build momentum for change. You can get into routines and rely on those routines to keep you going. Twisted ankles, bad backs, flus, colds, and other problems can kill momentum by changing your routines.

Aggressive management of injuries and illnesses can preserve momentum for effective weight control. For example, one of my clients, David, developed chronic sinus infections after the birth of his second child. Children bring a lot of joy into life—but a lot of colds as well. David had allergy problems, but his children's "gift" of frequent colds increased his problems. Sinus infections are like mild colds that also produce fevers and sluggishness. Unfortunately, they don't go away in seven days. They tend to stick around for weeks or months, if untreated by antibiotics. David found it difficult to maintain his jogging program, and thereby control his weight, because of these sinus infections.

He went to see an ear, nose, and throat specialist and an allergist. After a variety of tests, David and his doctors decided that the best course of action for him was to use very strong doses of antibiotics. He was to take this medicine as soon as he felt a new sinus infection beginning.

Last year, David got his usual dose of four or five sinus infections. But unlike the previous year, in which these infections greatly interfered with his life, this year each time an infection began, the antibiotics let him feel pretty good after just two days. So last year he was sick for approximately eight to ten days, instead of eight to ten weeks, as in the previous year.

Other clients have pursued alternative exercises when illness, sprained ankles, or back problems interfered with their usual routines. Exercycling puts a lot less pressure on backs, and sometimes less on knees, than walking or running. These are challenging transitions, but they are also inevitable. Successful weight controllers become, essentially, athletes. Athletes push their bodies hard. Successful weight controllers push their bodies hard as well.

Many times physicians and other specialists can help. But these helpers can also be quite frustrating. They offer solutions that sometimes don't work. Some solutions produce side effects that are worse than the problem. Searching for effective solutions might involve going from one health-care professional to another until you find the right approach. Knee and back problems are notorious for this kind of frustration. Sometimes physical therapists can help; sometimes orthopedic surgeons can help; sometimes chiropractors can help. Successful weight controllers keep trying until they find something that works. They also accept frustration as one of the more unpleasant results of doing what has to be done to remain successful.

In sum, to manage your injuries and illnesses effectively:

- Be aggressive about seeking help when needed.
- Expect frustration when seeking help.
- Find alternative means of exercising as soon as possible when injuries or illnesses interfere with your usual routines.

Scale Phobia

"I don't want to get on a scale this week because I think I gained weight." Does this sound familiar? It's a problematic attitude that can lead to relapsing.

Scales provide necessary information to weight controllers. If you avoid getting on a scale because you think you may have gained weight, you begin a pattern of avoiding self-monitoring. Remember, when people discontinue self-monitoring, they often discontinue effective self-control. Scales do not make judgments; only people can judge themselves. If you see a number that is higher than you'd like, you can do something about it. Avoiding the number on the scale just reinforces avoidance of the problem. *If you avoid this problem, it never goes away.*

Remember, your biology takes no vacations and cuts you no slack. You can try to make a deal with your biology, such as "If I don't look at the consequences of what you do to me, will you be kinder and gentler toward me?" Your fat cells will answer, "No way! I just want to get filled up. I don't care when or how or what it takes to get me filled up. I just want fat."

The best way to kill a scale phobia is to get on the scale. You can simply commit to weighing yourself at least once a week and dealing with whatever number you see. A very large study conducted by Weight Watchers showed that people who maintained their weight successfully for one year or more used a three-pound window. That is, successful weight controllers in the Weight Watchers program observed their weight carefully. When they noticed that they had gained as much as three pounds, they aggressively focused on their eating and exercising again to bring the weight back down immediately. Their less successful counterparts, people who regained substantial amounts of weight within a year after losing it, used a ten-pound window. These individuals paid much less attention to their weight. They allowed their weight to fluctuate by as much as ten pounds. They obviously had a more difficult time bringing their weight back down to more acceptable levels after they had gained as much as ten pounds.

It helps to use a narrow weight window and to continue weighing yourself regularly every week. You might find it useful to keep a graph of your weight. Perhaps you could hang it on the inside of your closet. You can write down the date you weighed yourself and your weight. You can look at this graph every day when you're getting your clothes and think about what it means.

Permanent Vacations

Most people find vacations relaxing, distracting, and enjoyable. Vacations are also dangerous to weight controllers. Vacations interfere with momentum. Vacations, like illnesses and injuries, cause changes in your usual routines. Renee, one of my clients, said, "I get into a 'vacation mentality.' The vacation mentality allows me to relax my restraint. I take it easy on myself. I don't force myself to exercise or count calories. I focus on my family and have fun." You can see that a "vacation mentality" can become a dangerous thing. Vacations can lead to decreases in exercise and re-emergence of higher-fat, higher-sugar eating. Once these patterns re-emerge, they become hard to kill off again.

People in the Acceptance stage find a way of treating vacations as opportunities for increased exercise and a vacation from their own refrigerators and cupboards. These individuals seek out exercise whenever possible during vacations and they know it will be easier to resist snacking on vacation. In fact, people in the Acceptance stage become "aggressively self-protective" and find vacations perfect opportunities to take good care of themselves. You can relax and have fun without high-fat, high-sugar eating and sedentary living.

Changes in Key Relationships

Major conflicts in key relationships can interfere with your life more dramatically than almost anything else. What happened to you the last time you had a major conflict at work? Most people report trouble sleeping and tremendous preoccupation when such conflicts occur. Conflicts at home produce even more dramatic symptoms. Major lapses can quickly become relapses during a period of conflict with friends, coworkers, and loved ones. The sense of "nothing else matters" can make effective eating and exercising seem absolutely trivial during these difficult times.

People almost always survive major conflicts with people who are significant and very important to them. Yet when these conflicts occur, your very survival can seem threatened. Conflicts, however, are normal parts of life. Millions of people have divorced and had huge upheavals in their jobs. And they have survived.

Survival tactics include obtaining support from friends during these difficult times. Exercise can help you relieve tensions. Eating high-fat and high-sugar foods may feel calming for a few minutes, but increased tension usually follows. Some weight controllers find it helpful to join Weight Watchers or a professional program during extreme periods of stress, such as those involving conflicts in relationships. If you take steps during conflicts to keep your weight-control efforts a high priority, you can maintain your momentum even during such difficult upheavals.

Work or Financial Crises

Losing a job or suffering major financial problems can interfere substantially with weight control. These crises, like crises in personal relationships, can make weight control seem unimportant. I've heard many clients say, "How can I worry about the number of fat grams I eat when my world is crumbling around me?"

Part of the answer to this question lies in the value of exercising regularly and following low-fat and low-sugar eating. Weight control certainly takes effort and focusing. Yet exercising effectively and eating in accord with a reasonable plan produces important benefits in your moods and feelings about yourself. *Weight control does not burden without benefit.* During a crisis on the job or a financial crisis, you can use weight control to provide stability and support in your life. If you view it this way, you may keep your exercising and eating patterns more effective than if you view weight control as a burden without any payoff. Eating foods that are high in sugar does, indeed, provide some immediate tranquilizing effects. This is part of what draws people to candy bars and other "goodies" during difficult times. It may also relieve some biological stress to decrease exercising or to relax your usual restraints about style of eating during such crises. However, increased weight and increased guilt may make such major lapses hardly worth their temporary benefits.

Consider working as aggressively as possible to solve both work and financial problems when they occur. Get help from friends and advisers about these situations. Begin networking to find another job, or take other steps to improve the job situation you are in. Remember that you are not on a diet. Your eating and exercising plan have become part of your life. Why give up an important and healthful part of your life just because another part of your life has gone awry?

Major Changes in Eating Environments

The following two stories show how major changes in environments can affect your eating patterns dramatically.

Arnie: "I got promoted a few months ago. I was really excited. It was a great opportunity. Unfortunately, it involved traveling two to three days per week. I figured, 'No big deal, I can handle this.' I didn't realize how much traveling around the country disrupted my usual routines. I found myself frustrated and irritated more of the time. Relaxation and cooling-out time became less and less. I felt tired in the morning and found it difficult to exercise at my usual time. I wound up in meetings in which all kinds of food (like muffins, doughnuts, pizza, cheese, and crackers) were carted in during all hours of the day and night. My eating and exercising habits began to break down, and I began gaining weight."

Jane: "I got a divorce last year. The time before the divorce was the real struggle (for about two years). The divorce was a tremendous relief for me. My weight was reasonably stable during the years before the divorce. I couldn't believe it, but I gained 20 pounds during this past year. It was such an adjustment. All of a sudden, for the first time in ten years, I was living by myself. I thought that would make it so much easier to control my food. I didn't realize that being in an unhappy relationship in some ways created fewer temptations for me than being alone. I found myself feeling lonely. Other times, I went out with friends to dinners and parties—far more often than I had in the last ten years. I was drinking more and eating bar food. I had more trouble sleeping, and that made it harder to get up early and exercise. I guess that's what did it."

As discussed in earlier chapters, traveling creates many challenges for weight controllers. Any substantial modification in your living situation also creates problems to be solved. Moving out of your house and into a college dormitory or moving out of a dormitory and into an apartment are transitions with which you are probably familiar. If you recall those transitions in your life, consider the impact they had on your eating and exercising. Have you ever heard of the "freshman 15"? Many college freshmen report gaining 15 pounds when they move into a college dormitory for the first time. These weight gains, while not documented scientifically, may occur for some people because of the tremendous changes in their usual routines.

If you experience such disruptions in your life, find a way to keep monitoring your weight and eating and exercising patterns; and if your weight and eating and exercising patterns begin to change in a problematic direction, take some steps to fix the problems. The latter point may include getting involved in a self-help or professional program, or it may include joining a health club. If you stay focused enough on this issue to observe the patterns of change in your eating, exercising, and weight, you will keep yourself in a position to handle changes effectively.

Poor Problem Solving

A recent study compared "maintainers" to "regainers." Maintainers were formerly obese women who had lost at least 20 pounds and maintained that loss for at least two years. Regainers were obese women who regained weight after losing at least 20 pounds. Regainers used "escape-avoidance" methods of solving problems much more so than did maintainers. These methods included eating, drinking, smoking, sleeping, and wishing the problems would just go away. Regainers also failed to get as much support from others ("social support") as did the maintainers. Most dramatically, maintainers reported confronting problems directly and aggressively, approximately ten times more frequently, than regainers. Successful weight controllers, both in this study and more generally, identify their problems quickly and then take action.

Abstinence Violation Effect (AVE)

Psychologists have identified a type of distortion in thinking that creates problems. The abstinence violation effect, or AVE, first involves making a commitment to abstinence. Many people who change their habits (for example, people who quit smoking or alcohol, as well as successful weight controllers) make a commitment to abstain forever from a certain pattern of eating or drinking. Weight controllers who do this may view themselves as "dieters."

What happens when a dieter eats a food that is not on the diet? For example, what happens when a dieter eats a piece of birthday cake? This dieter may view this initial lapse as a major conflict. The conflict might sound something like this in the mind of the dieter: "How can I be a dieter if I ate a piece of birthday cake?" One way of resolving this conflict is to abandon dieting. In other words, abstinence violation effects are relapses that occur to reduce the internal

conflict created by lapses. When weight controllers commit to unrealistically stringent standards for eating or exercising, they set the stage for AVEs. Following this commitment, initial lapses can produce major conflicts. These internal conflicts can be resolved by going into a full-blown relapse—"I can eat cake now because I am no longer a dieter."

You can avoid AVEs by adopting more realistic and reasonable goals. It makes no sense for weight controllers to commit to abstinence. Weight controllers simply cannot control their biologies and their situations perfectly. If you commit to abstaining from all sugar forever, you set yourself up for an AVE. How can you handle the initial lapse, the first ice cream cone or piece of cake, when you adopt such an unreasonable goal? It is critical to avoid placing yourself in such a conflict. Instead, it helps if you understand that weight controllers, even the most successful weight controllers, eat and exercise imperfectly. Lapses are inevitable. If you eat a problematic food, identify it as a lapse, write it down, and realize that a lapse, or two lapses, or a thousand lapses *do not make you any less of a weight controller*. You are an effective weight controller as long as you confront the issues involved with managing weight consistently and directly. You become a "nondieter" or "non–weight controller" only when you stick your head in the proverbial sand. When you refuse to get back on a scale or discontinue observing your eating and exercising, then and only then do you become a non–weight controller.

Slump Busters

Whether your slump was caused by an injury, illness, a scale phobia, a permanent vacation, or a major change in your relationships or eating environments, now what? The previous section, about the causes of slumps, also contained some ideas about how to deal with them. The following ideas add to those suggestions. You can see that all of them require action. Insight alone won't do it. Regaining momentum requires some notable action that leads to an even more notable change in your life. Consider using the following ideas to guide you toward that kind of active change: healthy obsession, health clubs, trainers, equipment, self-help, and professional help.

The Right Attitude: Healthy Obsession

When consistent exercisers stop exercising, even for one day, they get rather testy. Regular exercising is a positive obsession. That means that people get used to the feelings associated with exercising (like the "runner's high") and rely on these feelings to help them feel good.

That same healthy obsession applies to successful weight controllers. When weight controllers who are in the Acceptance stage find their usual routines of eating, exercising, and monitoring disrupted, they also get testy. These individuals have developed a healthy obsession with weight control. They rely on a certain approach to eating and exercising and observing themselves in order to feel comfortable. Disruptions are greeted with annoyance, irritability, and dissatisfaction. This is the attitude that defines successful weight controllers; it shows a very strong commitment to permanent weight control.

Some weight controllers become secretly happy when opportunities to stray from their usual patterns emerge. You may have noticed this in yourself or others. "Oh well, I was at a party and there was nothing else to eat—so I ate!" Those who adopt healthy obsessions about weight control hold themselves to a higher standard. They find it unacceptable to deviate from their plans without dealing with those deviations as problems. This doesn't mean that they berate themselves or abuse themselves when problems develop. It does mean that they see deviations as problems and attempt to deal with them directly. Wouldn't it be great if successful weight control meant having a happy-go-lucky attitude and feeling free of the oppression that seems required for success? It just doesn't work that way. The biology of excess weight is simply too tenacious. It takes a certain level of control, focusing, and intensity to manage it effectively.

Some of my clients who have lost a lot of weight and kept it off for years have lamented, "Now that I've lost all this weight, I expected to feel good about myself most of the time. But I don't. I still struggle with this every day." Sadly, this is the nature of the battle with the biology of excess weight. Most people do not view their own successes at weight control as joyous accomplishments. People who lose a lot of weight are typically less than thrilled about their new weight statuses. Usually, they want to lose another 5, 10, or 20 pounds. Even if they find their new weights acceptable, they still have to work hard to maintain their focusing. There may be a certain "joy in the discipline." Exercise can bring its own rewards, as can a sense of control about eating patterns. Nevertheless, the state in which many successful weight controllers find themselves feels more like "healthy obsession" than "joyous accomplishment."

Health Clubs

Many years ago health clubs were places for fanatics, weight lifters, grunters and groaners, and athletes. Now they serve as a social melting pot and meeting place. They also provide many comforts and a very wide range of activities, including low-impact and no-impact aerobic classes, spinning classes, water aerobics activities, yoga, instruction in almost every indoor sport imaginable, and machines, machines, machines. These centers of physical activity can serve as effective slump busters. When people join such centers, they tend to use them, at least for a while. Their novelty and the diversity of activities can motivate members to refocus on healthy eating and exercising.

When selecting a health club, keep in mind its three most important qualities: location, location, location! You will find that you actually use your health club when you either live very near it or work near it. If you belong to a health club located close to your house, you may use it in the morning. Almost all of the thousands of weight controllers with whom I have worked over the last twenty-five years, and who have succeeded at this difficult enterprise, have exercised primarily in the morning. Morning exercise proves most reliable because it interferes less in your daily life. After all, in the morning, you have complete control of your schedule and you can exercise before getting showered and dressed for the day. Exercising at any other time of the day requires taking a second shower and interrupting your activities. Yet another advantage of morning exercise concerns attitude. You may have noticed that you feel better during the day if you exercise first thing in the morning. For all of these reasons, consider choosing a health club near your home, if at all possible.

Trainers

Many people use trainers to help motivate them. Working with a trainer can help you learn about different types of equipment. For example, if you decide to begin a weight-lifting program, a trainer can provide important instruction on technique and help you set up an effective regimen. Trainers can also provide encouragement and support. Also, if you set up an appointment with a trainer, and particularly if you prepay for that appointment, you will motivate yourself to go, increasing your chances of doing some constructive exercising that day.

Try to find trainers who have advanced degrees in physical education or who are certified as athletic trainers. The American College of Sports Medicine certifies trainers. The world's largest certifier of trainers is the American Council on Exercise (ACE). ACE-certified trainers have passed a rigorous test demonstrating a detailed knowledge of physical exercise and conditioning principles. If you select a trainer who has an advanced degree in physical education and/or appropriate certification, you can feel more confident that the advice you get is grounded in science rather than hearsay. Unfortunately, personal trainers can cost from $10 to $100 per hour. Prices vary depending on standards used within the health club, training, and whether the trainers come to your house or you go to their facilities. If you are in a major slump, paying the price of weekly sessions with a personal trainer for a month or two may well be worth it.

Equipment

"I couldn't get myself focused until I bought a treadmill. It was a major expense (almost $2,000), but I get on that thing every day now. I really like it. I like having it in my house because of the flexibility and the reminder it provides. When I see it sitting there (which is very easy because it's huge), I know how important my weight-control efforts are to me." These sentiments were expressed by one of my former clients. She had indeed gotten into a major slump and was very excited about the way her new treadmill helped her get out of it.

An equipment purchase can prove very motivating for the reasons this former client outlined. Having the equipment in your home makes it much easier to exercise. Many people who have weight problems are reluctant to go to health clubs. They find the looks and comments of other people disconcerting. Of course, overweight people have as much right to use facilities at health clubs as any other customers. Yet the feelings can be so strong for some people that overcoming them is very difficult. Some people also live in climates that make outdoor exercising, such as walking or jogging, particularly challenging. These challenges can be overcome with appropriate clothing. However, when it's ten below zero or icy, you won't even find hardy souls merrily walking around outside.

Some very adequate exercycles are available for a few hundred dollars. More elaborate pieces of high-quality equipment, such as treadmills, carry much higher price tags. The best way to decide which piece of equipment makes the most sense for you is to go to a health club and try out the equipment. If you try out various pieces of equipment for several weeks, you will determine which kind is most comfortable for you and which you might use consistently.

Consumer Reports routinely evaluates exercise equipment for home use. Your local library includes copies of recent issues of *Consumer Reports*. The publisher of this magazine also prints books that summarize their findings. Before spending hundreds of dollars, perhaps thousands, consider studying the available evidence about which pieces of equipment work most effectively and reliably.

Self-Help Programs and Books

The long-term plan presented earlier in this chapter includes the possibility of participating in either Take Off Pounds Sensibly (TOPS) or Weight Watchers. These programs cost either nothing (TOPS) or relatively modest amounts of money (Weight Watchers). Every major city in the United States and many smaller towns have TOPS and Weight Watchers groups that meet frequently. These approaches provide support for change and may help you focus.

Many self-help books, videotapes, CDs, and computer programs can help you refocus. Information about relaxation, eating, nutrition, depression, visualization, or other topics may reawaken your commitment to effective weight control. The reference notes at the end of this book include titles on exercise, weight control, nutrition, and stress management.

Radical Changes in Diet

Radical changes in eating plans can sometimes break slumps. They require concentration, but they may serve as rallying points for change. Usually, radical dietary approaches suffer the same fate as all diets: They do not work for very long. But as a temporary step, making a major shift in your eating plan could spark important changes. You could try, for example, a vegetarian approach. Or you could eliminate bread and related foods.

Medications

Joe, a very obviously overweight middle-aged man, went to see his doctor about the new "diet" medications. "Doc," he said, "I've got to have those new meds that will get me to believe I just ate a turkey dinner."

"Well, Joe, I don't know about the turkey dinner part," his doctor answered, "but they could help you lose weight if you're willing to work at it."

"But Doc, I thought those pills made you feel like you just ate a turkey dinner and then they also made you really want to work at it."

"Sorry, Joe. For the turkey dinner, you have to go to a grocery store. To really want to work at it, you have to find that within yourself somewhere—not in your medicine cabinet."

Physicians began prescribing amphetamines (Benzedrine) more than fifty years ago to help people lose weight. Unfortunately, Benzedrine did more than reduce their appetites; it is an addictive drug that produces a "high" that people crave. Thousands of people became addicted to Benzedrine in an attempt to lose weight. That drug and others like it can no longer be prescribed in the United States or England for weight control. Prescriptions for those drugs are carefully monitored by governmental agencies.

Many physicians know this sad tale. They believe that any drug prescribed for weight control may cause more harm than good. This view, while understandable, no longer fits the current scientific information about medications for weight control. Despite the bias against them, some modern medications can help people decrease their appetite and feel full sooner. These efforts can occur with virtually no risk for causing addictions. Does this sound too good to be true?

Medications that help control appetite can also produce such side effects as depression, irritability, dizziness, insomnia, and nausea. The best of the medications produce very few of these effects for most people. However, these effects, when they do occur, can be quite annoying. Furthermore, the research on these medications suggests that they work while they are taken, but that soon after they are discontinued, even if they were taken for six months or a year, many people regain all of the weight they lost. And these medications generally produce small amounts of weight loss.

Modern medications for weight control still have an important role to play. First, if you take these medications while participating in an active weight-control program, they might really help you. I have seen this happen with many of my clients. Their weight losses had slowed down or stopped for various reasons. After they began a course of drug treatment, their eating and exercising improved markedly. I have seen quite a few people use the medications, lose 10 to 20 pounds, get off the medications, and continue to lose weight.

The medications popularly known as fen-phen (fenfluramine and phentermine, sometimes known as Pondimin and Ionamin) had been used for more than ten years. A related medication that was rather close in its effects to fenfluramine (Pondimin), Redux (dex-fenfluramine), was the first appetite-control medication approved by the Food and Drug Administration (FDA) in twenty-three years. Some recent case studies and some very expensive lawsuits led the manufacturers of both Pondimin and Redux to discontinue their availability in the fall of 1997. The scientific basis for this action was minimal. Now Ionamin is still available and can be prescribed with some close cousins to fenfluramine (for example, Paxil or Zoloft). The effectiveness of those combinations, however, has not been tested.

A newer medication, Meridia (sibutramine), acts like fen-phen and is the best available appetite-control medication. Medical monitoring by physicians who know these medications is necessary to maximize safety and effectiveness. Any drug can produce side effects, some rather troubling, and these medications are no exception.

Another medication (orlistat, sometimes called Xenical) contains an enzyme that blocks the absorption of fat, at least the absorption of about one-third of the fat consumed. Some preliminary research suggests that some people respond favorably to taking this medication and lose modest amounts of weight. However, if you follow the principles in this book (for example, eating as little fat as possible), orlistat will not prove helpful. In addition, most people will experience some notable and troublesome digestive problems associated with taking a medication that extracts fat from food (including flatulence, oily stools, and bloating). Successful weight controllers tend to find ways of eating low-fat foods and making that a permanent part of their lifestyles. Reliance on this medication for that purpose seems unlikely as an effective long-term strategy. On the other hand, it might be useful to use a medication like this on the occasions (rare, one hopes) when you do overeat high-fat foods. If taken within an hour of the problematic food or meal, it could decrease the impact of the fat.

It is critical to emphasize that it only makes sense to take these medications if you are participating in a professionally conducted weight-control program. Scientific research suggests that these medications produce few benefits unless weight controllers get help focusing on eating and exercising through a professional program while they are taking them.

If prescription medications for weight control can help some participants in professional programs, can over-the-counter drugs (such as Dexatrim and others) help anyone? Probably not. One of the two nonprescription drugs that are available in the United States, phenylpropanolamine (PPA), acts like a mild stimulant. PPA can produce some small weight losses, but the effects do not last long. PPA is found in most nonprescription "weight-control" drugs. Benzocaine, the other approved nonprescription drug, is found in some over-the-counter "appetite-suppressant" or "weight-control" drugs. By numbing your taste buds, it supposedly decreases your interest in food. It does not work.

If you want to try medications for weight control, first join a professional program. Then discuss this possibility with your therapist from that program and consider only prescription medications—if you and your therapist view that option as worthwhile.

Professional Help

Consumer Reports recently reported on the largest survey ever conducted of people who had obtained professional help for a variety of psychological problems. More than four thousand readers of that magazine answered twenty-six questions about mental-health professionals, family doctors, and support groups from which they'd sought help for psychological distress. Among their most intriguing, and hopeful, findings were:

- People who obtained help from their family doctors tended to feel better after obtaining the help. But people who saw a mental-health specialist for more than six months did *much better*.
- Most people who took medications for psychological problems (like Prozac or Xanax) reported feeling better, but about half of the respondents reported substantial and troublesome side effects (like drowsiness and a feeling of disorientation).
- The longer people stayed in therapy, the more they improved.
- Most people who went to a self-help group (like Alcoholics Anonymous) were very satisfied with the experience and said they got better.
- Almost everyone who sought help experienced some relief, but people who started out feeling the worst reported the most progress.

Mental-health professionals define depression as including at least five of the following problems for at least two weeks. At least one of the problems must be either (1) depressed mood or (2) loss of interest in pleasure:

1. Depressed mood, most of the day, nearly every day.

2. Markedly less interest or pleasure in all, or almost all, activities most of the day, nearly every day.

3. Significant weight loss or weight gain when not dieting, or increase in appetite nearly every day.

4. Insomnia or hypersomnia (excess sleeping) nearly every day.

5. Excess physical movement or slowing down in physical movements, nearly every day.

6. Fatigue or loss of energy every day.

7. Feelings of worthlessness or excessive or inappropriate guilt, nearly every day.

8. Decreased ability to think or concentrate, or indecisiveness, nearly every day.

9. Recurrent thoughts of death (not just fear of dying), recurrent suicidal thoughts without a suicide attempt or a specific plan for committing suicide.

Many people experience significant depressions and other forms of psychological distress at some points in their lives. You can imagine how depression can interfere with successful weight control. When feeling depressed, people struggle to stay focused on almost anything in their lives, let alone something as difficult as warding off the biology of excess weight. I have heard many people say, "I just didn't care." This statement often accompanies significant lapses or slumps. Unfortunately, once again, your biology has no sympathy. If you feel lousy, for whatever reason, your biology will be more than happy to add excess pounds.

People try many things to get out of depression and other unpleasant psychological states. You can try talking to close friends, taking vacations, or changing something significant in your life. When all of your best efforts do not produce positive change, consider taking the next step. You can seek professional help for marital problems or problems with your moods, such as depression. You can ask close friends or relatives for referrals to licensed professionals in your area whom they know or have heard good things about. You can also call your local hospital or university and ask how to get professional assistance.

Most health-insurance policies cover substantial amounts of the costs involved with such treatment. Most communities also provide relatively low-cost counseling. You can find these services by calling your church or synagogue or your local mental-health association.

If at all possible, try to find a therapist who is licensed in your state and is either a psychologist, a social worker, or a psychiatrist. Psychologists receive five to eight years of training beyond a bachelor's degree. This training focuses on the scientific aspects of helping people change. Social workers receive one to three years of training beyond a bachelor's degree, focused on how to form good relationships with people and how to use community resources that can prove helpful. Psychiatrists receive a medical degree and then several years of training beyond that, specializing in how to help people with significant problems in their lives.

Psychiatrists are the only mental-health professionals who can prescribe medications. However, this may not be an advantage. Most psychiatrists prescribe medications too quickly. You can find yourself being treated with a powerful set of medications (sometimes with complicated side effects) while other, less chemical, methods could have produced better outcomes. Therefore, I recommend seeing a licensed psychologist or social worker before seeing a psychiatrist. If these other licensed mental-health professionals feel that medications could be helpful to you, they will certainly recommend that you get a consultation from a psychiatrist in order to use such treatments. I believe that if you can find a way of changing without using medications, you will achieve better results and feel better in the long run.

Many weight controllers who become depressed delay getting help. Certainly problems take a while to resolve on your own. You may ask friends or family members for help. You may read about the problem and attempt to change yourself. These efforts are worthy of admiration and respect. If and when they do not produce positive outcomes, however, please take action quickly. Your biology acts very quickly to cause you trouble. A lapse quickly turns into a slump or a relapse. To avoid this downward spiral, *action* must become your middle name. Your biology does not allow you to stay in a slump very long without punishing you much more severely than the person who doesn't struggle with weight problems.

Sports psychologists provide very similar advice to elite athletes. When athletes struggle with emotional issues, their performances decline, just as your weight increases. Performance declines can rapidly become major slumps. Major slumps can ruin careers. Athletes, and weight controllers, must take action quickly to grapple with whatever problems face them. Quick action on the part of athletes can end slumps. The same applies to you.

"Let us run with endurance the race that is set before us."
—Hebrews 12:1

Reference Sources

Chapter One

Eckel, R. H. (1989). "Lipoprotein Lipase: A Multifunctional Enzyme Relevant to Common Metabolic Diseases." *New England Journal of Medicine,* 320: 1060–68.

Johnson, W. G., and H. E. Wildman (1983). "Influence of External and Covert Food Stimuli on Insulin Secretion in Obese and Normal Persons." *Behavioral Neuroscience,* 97: 1025–28.

Kirschenbaum, D. S. (1987). "Self-Regulatory Failure: A Review with Clinical Implications." *Clinical Psychology Review,* 7: 77–104.

Kirschenbaum, D. S. (1994). *Weight Loss through Persistence: Making Science Work for You.* Oakland, Calif.: New Harbinger Publications.

Kirschenbaum, D. S., and P. Karoly (1977). "When Self-Regulation Fails: Tests of Some Preliminary Hypotheses." *Journal of Consulting and Clinical Psychology,* 45: 1116–25.

Mantzoros, C. S. (1999). "The Role of Leptin in Human Obesity and Disease: A Review of Current Evidence." *Annals of Internal Medicine,* 130: 671–80.

McGuire, M. T., R. R. Wing, M. L. Klem, W. Lang, and J. O. Hill (1999). "Behavioral Strategies of Individuals Who Have Maintained Long-Term Weight Losses." *Obesity Research,* 7: 334–41.

McGuire, M. T., R. R. Wing, M. L. Klem, W. Lang, and J. O. Hill (1999). "What Predicts Weight Regain in a Group of Successful Weight Losers?" *Journal of Consulting and Clinical Psychology,* 67: 177–85.

Meichenbaum, D., and D. C. Turk (1987). *Facilitating Treatment Adherence: A Practitioner's Guidebook.* New York: Plenum.

Perri, M. G., A. M. Nezu, and B. J. Viegener (1992). *Improving the Long-Term Management of Obesity: Theory, Research and Clinical Guidelines.* New York: John Wiley.

Ravussin, E., and B. A. Swinburn (1993). "Energy Metabolism." In A. J. Stunkard and T. A. Wadden, eds., *Obesity: Theory and Therapy.* 2nd ed. New York: Raven Press.

Staff writer (1996). "Weight-Loss News That's Easy to Stomach." *Tufts University Diet and Nutrition Letter,* p. 14.

Stunkard, A. J. (1958). "The Management of Obesity." *New York State Journal of Medicine,* 58: 79–87.

Vincent, P. (1971). "Factors Influencing Patient Noncompliance: A Theoretical Approach." *Nursing Research,* 20: 509–16.

Wadden, T. A. (1993). "Treatment of Obesity by Moderate and Severe Caloric Restriction: Results of Clinical Research Trials." *Annals of Internal Medicine,* 119: 688–93.

Chapter Two

Hubbel, M. A., B. L. Duncan, and S. D. Miller, eds. (1999). *The Heart and Soul of Change: What Works in Therapy.* Washington, D.C.: American Psychological Association.

Ikemi, Y., and S. Nakagawa (1962). "A Psychosomatic Study of Contagious Dermatitis." *Kyosu Journal of Medical Science,* 13: 335–50.

Kirsch, I. (1990). *Changing Expectations: A Key to Effective Psychotherapy.* Pacific Grove, Calif.: Brooks/Cole.

Kirschenbaum, D. S., M. L. Fitzgibbon, S. Martino, J. H. Conviser, E. H. Rosendahl, and L. Laatsch (1992). "Stages of Change in Successful Weight Control: A Clinically Derived Model." *Behavior Therapy,* 23: 623–35.

Nelson, L. R., and M. L. Furst (1972). "An Objective Study of the Effects of Expectation on Competitive Performance." *Journal of Psychology,* 81: 69–72.

Shapiro, A. K. (1978). "Placebo Effects in Medicine, Psychotherapy, and Psychoanalysis." In A. P. Bergin and S. L. Garfield, eds., *Handbook of Psychotherapy and Behavior Change: An Empirical Analysis.* New York: John Wiley.

Chapter Three

Banting, W. (1863). "Letter on Corpulence, Addressed to the Public." Kensington, England: Published by the author.

Bessesen, D. H., C. L. Rupp, and R. H. Eckel (1995). "Dietary Fat Is Shunted Away from Oxidation, Towards Storage in Obese Zucker Rats." *Obesity Research,* 3: 179–89.

Blass, E. (1989). "Opioids, Sweets, and a Mechanism for Positive Affect: Broad

Motivational Implications." In J. Dobbing, ed., *Sweetness*. New York: Springer-Verlag.

Blundell, J. E., V. J. Burley, J. R. Cotton, and C. L. Lawton (1993). "Dietary Fat in the Control of Energy Intake: Evaluating the Effects of Fat on Meal Size and Postmeal Satiety." *American Journal of Clinical Nutrition*, 57: 772S–78S.

Boozer, C. N., A. Brasseur, and R. L. Atkinson, (1993). "Dietary Fat Affects Weight Loss and Adiposity during Energy Restriction in Rats." *American Journal of Clinical Nutrition*, 58: 846–52.

Brody, J. (1987). *Jane Brody's Nutrition Book*. New York: Bantam Books.

Cohler, S. (1988). "Food for Thought." *Psychology Today*, p. 30.

Dobbing, J., ed. (1987). *Sweetness*. New York: Springer-Verlag.

Geiselman, P. J., and D. Novin (1982). "The Role of Carbohydrates in Appetite, Hunger and Obesity." *Appetite*, 3: 203–23.

Hill, J. O., H. Drougas, and J. C. Peters (1993). "Obesity Treatment: Can Diet Composition Play a Role?" *Annals of Internal Medicine*, 119: 694–97.

Jeffery, R. W., W. L. Hellerstedt, S. A. French, and J. E. Baxter (1995). "A Randomized Trial of Counseling for Fat Restriction versus Calorie Restriction in the Treatment of Obesity." *International Journal of Obesity*, 19: 132–37.

Netzer, C. T. (1991). *The Complete Book of Food Counts*. 2nd ed. New York: Dell Publishing.

Sims, E. Z. H., E. Danforth, et al. (1973). "Endocrine and Metabolic Effects of Experimental Obesity in Man." *Recent Progress in Hormone Research*, 29: 457–87.

Staff writers (December 1998). "Diet and Cancer: The Big Picture." *Nutrition Action Health Letter*, 25: 10.

Staff writers (December 1998). "Seven Excuses for Not Eating Better (That Don't Hold Up Under Close Scrutiny)." *Tufts University Health and Nutritional Letter*.

Thayer, R. E. (1987). "Energy, Tiredness, and Tension Effects of a Sugar Snack versus Moderate Exercise." *Journal of Personality and Social Psychology*, 52: 119–25.

Van Horn, L., and R. E. Kaevey (1997). "Diet and Cardiovascular Disease Prevention: What Works?" *Annals of Behavioral Medicine*, 19: 197–212.

Chapter Four

Baker, R. C., and D. S. Kirschenbaum (1993). "Self-Monitoring May Be Necessary for Successful Weight Control." *Behavior Therapy* 24: 377–94.

Baker, R. C., and D. S. Kirschenbaum (1998). "Weight Control during the Holidays: Highly Consistent Self-Monitoring as a Potentially Useful Coping Mechanism." *Health Psychology*, 17: 367–70.

Baumeister, R. F., T. F. Heatherton, and D. M. Tice (1994). *Losing Control: How and Why People Fail at Self-Regulation.* San Diego: Academic Press.

Boutelle, K. N., and D. S. Kirschenbaum (1998). "Further Support for Consistent Self-Monitoring as a Vital Component of Successful Weight Control." *Obesity Research,* 6: 219–24.

Boutelle, K. N., D. S. Kirschenbaum, R. C. Baker, and M. E. Mitchell (1999). "How Can Obese Weight Controllers Minimize Weight Gain During the High Risk Holiday Season? By Self-Monitoring Very Consistently." *Health Psychology,* 18: 364–68.

Carver, C. S., and M. F. Scheier (1990). "Origins and Functions of Positive and Negative Affect: A Control-Process View." *Psychological Review,* 97: 19–35.

Kanfer, F. H., and P. Karoly (1972). "Self-Control: A Behavioristic Excursion into the Lion's Den." *Behavior Therapy,* 3: 398–416.

Kirschenbaum, D. S. (1987). "Self-Regulatory Failure: A Review with Clinical Implications." *Clinical Psychology Review,* 7: 77–104.

Perri, M. G., A. M. Nezu, and B. J. Viegener (1992). *Improving the Long-Term Management of Obesity: Theory, Research, and Clinical Guidelines.* New York: John Wiley.

Schlundt, D. G., T. Sbrocco, and C. Bell (1989). "Identification of High Risk Situations in a Behavioral Weight Loss Program: Application of the Relapse Prevention Model." *International Journal of Obesity,* 13: 223–34.

Sperduto, W. A., H. S. Thompson, and R. M. O'Brien (1986). "The Effect of Target Behavior Monitoring on Weight Loss and Completion Rate in a Behavior Modification Program for Weight Reduction." *Addictive Behaviors,* 11: 337–40.

Weinberg, R. S. (1988). *The Mental Advantage: Developing Your Psychological Skills in Tennis.* Champaign, Ill.: Leisure Press.

Chapter Five

Baechle, T. R., and B. R. Groves (1992). *Weight Training: Steps to Success.* Champaign, Ill.: Leisure Press.

Blair, S. N. (1991). *Living with Exercise.* Dallas: American Health Publishing.

Blair, S. N. (1991). "Weight Loss through Physical Activity." *Weight Control Digest,* 1: 17, 20–24.

Curless, M. R. (September 1992). "Only the Fit Stay Young." *Self,* pp. 180–81.

Dishman, R. K., ed. (1988). *Exercise Adherence: Its Impact on Public Health.* Champaign, Ill.: Human Kinetics Publishers.

Donahoe, C. P., Jr., D. H. Lin, D. S. Kirschenbaum, and R. E. Keesey (1984). "Metabolic Consequences of Dieting and Exercise in the Treatment of Obesity." *Journal of Consulting and Clinical Psychology,* 52: 827–36.

Galvin, J. (1991). *The Exercise Habit: Your Personal Road Map to Developing a Lifelong Exercise Commitment.* Champaign, Ill.: Human Kinetics Publishers.

Heil, J. (1993). *Psychology of Sport Injury.* Champaign, Ill.: Human Kinetics Publishers.

Kendzierski, D., and W. Johnson (1993). "Excuses, Excuses, Excuses: A Cognitive Behavioral Approach to Exercise Implementation." *Journal of Sport and Exercise Psychology,* 15: 207–19.

Kirschenbaum, D. S. (1998). *Mind Matters: Seven Steps to Smarter Sport Performance.* Carmel, Ind.: Cooper Publishing Group.

Kusinitz, I., M. Fin, and the Editors of Consumer Reports Books (1983). *Physical Fitness for Practically Everybody: The Consumers Union Report on Exercise.* Mount Vernon, N.Y.: Consumers Union.

Latella, F. S., W. Conkling, and the Editors of Consumer Reports Books (1989). *Get in Shape, Stay in Shape.* Mount Vernon, N.Y.: Consumer Reports Books.

Rippe, J. M., and P. Amend (1992). *The Exercise Exchange Program.* New York: Simon & Schuster.

Vickery, S., and M. Moffat (1999). *The American Physical Therapy Association Book of Body Repair and Maintenance.* New York: Owl Books.

Chapter Six

Alberti, R. E., and M. L. Emmons (1990). *Your Perfect Right: A Guide to Assertive Living.* 6th ed. San Luis Obispo, Calif.: Impact Publishers.

American Psychiatric Association (1987). *Diagnostic and Statistical Manual of Mental Disorders.* 3rd ed., rev. Washington, D.C.: American Psychiatric Association.

Barlow, D.H., and R. M. Rapee (1991). *Mastering Stress: A Lifestyle Approach.* Dallas: American Health Publishing.

Beckfield, D. F. (1994). *Master Your Panic and Take Back Your Life!* San Luis Obispo, Calif.: Impact Publishers.

Bernstein, D. A., and D. T. Borkovec (1973). *Progressive Relaxation Training: A Manual for the Helping Professions.* Champaign, Ill.: Research Press.

Birkedahl, N. (1991). *Older and Wiser: A Workbook for Coping with Aging.* Oakland, Calif.: New Harbinger Publications.

Bourne, E. J. (1990). *The Anxiety and Phobia Workbook.* Oakland, Calif.: New Harbinger Publications.

Burns, D. E. (1989). *The Feeling Good Handbook: Using the New Mood Therapy in Everyday Life.* New York: William Morrow.

Cautela, J. R., and J. Groden (1991). *Relaxation: A Comprehensive Manual for Adults, Children, and Children with Special Needs.* Champaign, Ill.: Research Press.

Davis, M., E. R. Eshelman, and M. McKay (1995). *The Relaxation and Stress Reduction Workbook*. 4th ed. Oakland, Calif.: New Harbinger Publications.

Grasha, A. F., and D. S. Kirschenbaum (1986). *Adjustment and Competence: Concepts and Applications*. Minneapolis: West Publishing.

Harp, D., with N. Feldman (1990). *The New Three Minute Mediator*. Oakland, Calif.: New Harbinger Publications.

Holmes, T. H., and R. H. Rahe (1967). "The Social Readjustment Rating Scale." *Journal of Psychosomatic Research,* 11: 216.

Jacobson, E. (1929). *Progressive Relaxation*. Chicago: University of Chicago Press.

Kirschenbaum, D. S. (1998). "Using Sport Psychology to Improve Health Psychology Outcomes." *The Health Psychologist,* 20: 16–17, 22–23.

Kirschenbaum, D. S., and D. A. Wittrock (1990). "Still Searching for Effective Criticism Inoculation Procedures." *Journal of Applied Sport Psychology,* 2: 175–85.

Kobasa, S. C., S. R. Maddi, and S. Kahn (1982). "Hardiness and Health: A Prospective Study." *Journal of Personality and Social Psychology,* 42:168–77.

Klarreich, S. H. (1990). *Work with Stress: A Practical Guide to Emotional Well-Being on the Job*. New York: Brunner/Mazel.

Marks, I. M. (1978). *Living with Fear: Understanding and Coping with Anxiety*. New York: McGraw-Hill.

McKay, M., and P. Fanning (1993). *Time Out from Stress*. (Two ten-minute cassettes.) Oakland, Calif.: New Harbinger Publications.

Meichenbaum, D. (1985). *Stress Inoculation Training*. New York: Pergamon.

Paine, W. S., ed. (1982). *Job Stress and Burnout*. Beverly Hills: Sage Publications.

Stevens, J. O. (1971). *Awareness: Exploring, Experimenting, Experiencing*. Moab, Utah: Real People Press.

Tubesing, N. L., and D. H. Tubesing (1990). *Structured Exercises in Stress Management*. Vols. 1–4. Duluth, Minn.: Whole Person Press.

Zilberg, N. J., D. S. Weiss, and M. J. Horowitz (1982). "Impact of Event Scale: A Cross-Validation Study." *Journal of Consulting and Clinical Psychology,* 50: 407–14.

Chapter Seven

Bray, G. A. (1995). "Pharmacologic Treatment of Obesity." *Obesity Research,* 3, supp. 4.

Greenway, G. (1992). "Non-prescription Medications for Weight Control: A Review." *American Journal of Clinical Nutrition,* 55: 203–5.

Ellis, A., and R. A. Harper (1975). *A New Guide to Rational Living*. North Hollywood, Calif.: Wilshire Book Co.

Kirschenbaum, D. S. (1992). "Elements of Effective Weight Control Programs: Implications for Exercise and Sport Psychology." *Journal of Applied Sport Psychology,* 4: 77–93.

Kirschenbaum, D. S. (1988). "Treating Adult Obesity in 1988: Evolution of a Modern Program." *The Behavior Therapist,* 11: 3–6.

Kirschenbaum, D. S., and A. J. Tomarken (1982). "On Facing the Generalization Problem: The Study of Self-Regulatory Failure." In P. C. Kendall, ed., *Advances in Cognitive-Behavioral Research and Therapy.* Vol. 1. New York: Academic Press.

Marlatt, G. A., and J. R. Gordon, eds. (1985). *Relapse Prevention: Maintenance Strategies in the Treatment of Addictive Behaviors.* New York: Guilford Press.

National Institutes of Health (1992). *Methods for Voluntary Weight Loss and Control: Technology Assessment Conference Statement.* Bethesda, Md.: NIH. (Available from: Office of Medical Applications of Research, NIH, Federal Building, Room 618, Bethesda, MD 10892).

Stunkard, A. J. (1958). "The Management of Obesity." *New York State Journal of Medicine,* 58: 79–87.

Stunkard, A. J., and T. A. Wadden, eds. (1983). *Obesity: Theory and Therapy.* 2nd ed. New York: Raven Press.

Wadden, T. A., and T. B. VanItallie, eds. (1992). *Treatment of the Seriously Obese Patient.* New York: Guilford Press.

Index